T0180221

Handbook of Neurocritical Care

CURRENT CLINICAL NEUROLOGY

Daniel Tarsy, MD, SERIES EDITOR

Handbook
of Neurocritical Care

Edited by

Anish Bhardwaj, MD

Marek A. Mirski, MD, PhD

John A. Ulatowski, MD, PhD, MBA

*Neurosciences Critical Care Unit, Johns Hopkins Hospital,
Johns Hopkins University School of Medicine*

Foreword by

Thomas P. Bleck, MD, FCCM

*Louise Nerancy Eminent Scholar in Neurology,
Professor of Neurology, Neurological Surgery, and Internal Medicine,
Director, Neuroscience Intensive Care Unit,
The University of Virginia,
President, The Neurocritical Care Society*

HUMANA PRESS ✳ TOTOWA, NEW JERSEY

Additional material to this book can be downloaded from http://extras.springer.com

Cover design by Patricia F. Cleary.

Production Editor: Tracy Catanese

For additional copies, pricing for bulk purchases, and/or information about other Humana titles, contact Humana at the above address or at any of the following numbers: Tel.: 973-256-1699; Fax: 973-256-8314; E-mail: humana@humanapr.com, or visit our Website: http://humanapress.com

Photocopy Authorization Policy:

Authorization to photocopy items for internal or personal use, or the internal or personal use of specific clients, is granted by Humana Press Inc., provided that the base fee of US $25.00 per copy is paid directly to the Copyright Clearance Center at 222 Rosewood Drive, Danvers, MA 01923. For those organizations that have been granted a photocopy license from the CCC, a separate system of payment has been arranged and is acceptable to Humana Press Inc. The fee code for users of the Transactional Reporting Service is: [0-58829-273-8/04 $25.00].

10 9 8 7 6 5 4 3 2

ISBN 1-59259-772-6 (eBook)

Library of Congress Cataloging in Publication Data

Handbook of neurocritical care / edited by Anish Bhardwaj, Marek A. Mirski, John A. Ulatowski.
    p. ; cm. -- (Current clinical neurology)
  Includes bibliographical references and index.
  ISBN 1-58829-273-8   ISBN 1-58829-078-6
  1. Neurological intensive care--Handbooks, manuals, etc.
  [DNLM: 1. Nervous System Diseases--therapy--Handbooks. 2. Critical Care--methods--Handbooks. 3. Intensive Care
Units--Handbooks. WL 39 H23663 2004] I. Bhardwaj, Anish. II. Mirski, Marek Alexander Z. III. Ulatowski, John Alan. IV. Series.
  RC350.N49H36 2004
  616.8'0428--dc22
                                                                2004005193

Series Editor's Introduction

The diagnosis and management of patients with critical neurologic and neurosurgical disorders has come a long way since the classic monograph Stupor and Coma by Plum and Posner was published in the early 1970s. Whereas that work emphasized diagnosis, the explosion of scientific and technological advances that impacts the management of critically ill patients has resulted in several texts in critical care neurology and neurosurgery, including the recent Current Clinical Series monograph, Critical Care Neurology and Neurosurgery by Suarez and colleagues. The Handbook of Neurocritical Care by Dr. Bhardwaj and his colleagues has now arrived to provide a handy, self-contained, and comprehensive guide that clinicians will find invaluable in the day-to-day care of patients with critical neurologic and neurosurgical illnesses.

The editors have assembled a highly qualified and respected group of critical care specialists who cover the field concisely but thoroughly. Importantly, nearly all of the contributors are multidisciplinary colleagues in neurology, neurosurgery, anesthesiology, and critical care medicine and nursing at the Johns Hopkins Hospitals, thereby providing a consistent approach to the management of these patients. Uniquely, this book provides a CD-ROM containing an eBook version of the volume that can be downloaded and viewed on a computer or handheld PDA. The Key Points and selected references provided at the end of each chapter provide easy access to essential information likely to be used in a setting where timely decision making is a critical element of treatment. Each chapter is marked by an orderly flow of information presented with easy-to-follow bullet points and tables. In addition to the chapters covering specific disease entities, the disciplines of neurological, neurosurgical, pulmonary, cardiovascular, cerebrovascular, and infectious disease management, anesthesia, neuromonitoring, neuropharmacology, nutrition, and bioethics are all covered in detail. This handbook covers the state-of-the-art concisely and completely and should become an integral part of the critical care unit armamentarium for the management of critically ill neurologic and neurosurgical patients.

Daniel Tarsy, MD
Chief, Movement Disorders Center
Department of Neurology
Beth Israel Deaconess Medical Center
Associate Professor of Neurology
Harvard Medical School

v

Foreword

Neurocritical care is simultaneously one of the oldest and newest aspects of medicine. The goals of neurocritical care date back at least to the 16th century, the time of Paracelsus, who introduced the concept of resuscitation. However, the modern threads of neurocritical care begin with neurosurgical work of MacEwen and Hutchinson in the 19th century, and Cushing in the 20th. Parallel developments in mechanical ventilation led to the first large-scale use of this technique in the poliomyelitis epidemics of the first half of the 20th century, when neurologists were the physicians for patients with ventilatory failure, and the nurses for these patients were the first critical care practitioners. The concept of an intensive care unit based on the advantages of concentrating the care of the sickest patients, rather than on a particular device, begins with Peter Safar at the Baltimore city hospital in 1963. These three distinct threads were combined in the United States by Michael Earnest at the University of Colorado in the late 1960s, and then brought into their present form by Allan Ropper, Sean Kennedy, and Nicholas Zervas at the Massachusetts General Hospital in the early 1970s. In the 1980s, similarly functioning units arose at Columbia University in New York, the Johns Hopkins Hospital in Baltimore, and the University of Virginia in Charlottesville. Now neurocritical care is expanding, with over 25 training programs in North America and many more worldwide. The discipline of neurocritical care is clearly coming into its own.

Critical care holds tremendous promise to improve patient outcomes and medical training. Several studies now document that instituting an intensivist-led multiprofessional team model for the care of critically ill patients produces improvements in survival, functional outcome, and expenses. Two studies, including one authored by a contributor to this book, show that care by specially trained neurointensivists is especially important for patients with nervous system disorders who require critical care.

The neurointensivist requires all of the skills expected of the general intensivist, and in addition must add the interpretive and management skills developed by training as clinical neuroscientists. As with any intensivist, the responsibilities of the neurointensivist extend beyond the care of the individual patient to the other aspects of running an intensive care unit, such as infection control, resource utilization, and personnel management. This more global view is one of the points by which the intensivist model adds more than just special expertise in the care of these vulnerable patients, thereby helping to improve outcomes for all of the patients in the unit simultaneously. The *Handbook of Neurocritical Care* provides a wealth of ideas and experience in many of these areas, and is a valuable resource for all physicians from the beginning resident to the seasoned intensive care unit director.

Neurocritical care nurses are also a special breed. Among the branches of critical care nursing, all of which are vital to the care of the critically ill, they

vii

have raised the standards of physical examination of their patients to new heights. The *Handbook of Neurocritical Care* should also be useful for them, whether they are in a setting in which they work with and teach house officers or work in institutions where they must function more independently.

One mark of the increasing maturity of neurocritical care is the recent creation of a professional organization uniting neurointensivists, neurocritical care nurses, neurosurgeons, and interventional neuro-radiologists. This Neurocritical Care Society recently held its second annual meeting, at which several contributors to the *Handbook of Neurocritical Care* presented papers. Some of the contributors also serve on the board of directors and committees of the Society. The interactions of various professions within the Society mirror the day-to-day coopera-tion and collaboration which characterizes the intensive care units in which they work. The new journal of the Society, *Neurocritical Care*, shares the same publisher as this text, demonstrating the commitment that Humana has made to the development of this field.

Over the past 15 years of growth of the discipline, I have had the privilege of knowing all of the contributors, and participating in research and education endeavors with several of them. Some have been active for many years, and others have recently completed their formal training. All of them are accomplished clinicians who impart their knowledge, wisdom, and experience in this text.

Despite the proven advantages of the intensivist-led model in general, and of neurointensivists for this patient population, the dramatic shortage of intensivists and critical care nurses limits the number of institutions who can adopt this model. For physicians and nurses practicing in these environments, a book such as this one provides quick access to the essen-tial aspects of diagnosis and management their patients need.

The design of the *Handbook of Neurocritical Care* makes the knowledge and wisdom it contains rapidly accessible. I believe it will find a place in many intensive care units, and hope that a copy will be available wherever clinicians need ready access to this information.

The contributors to this handbook are all connected to the neurocritical care service of Johns Hopkins in some manner. They have built one of the world's premier research, training, and clinical programs in the field, and a snapshot of their experience is summarized here. This field is growing rapidly, and there will undoubtedly be a need for frequent editions of this text at the leading edge of knowledge.

Thomas P. Bleck, MD, FCCM
Louise Nerancy Eminent Scholar in Neurology, Professor
of Neurology, Neurological Surgery, and Internal Medicine,
Director, Neuroscience Intensive Care Unit,
The University of Virginia
President (2003–2005), The Neurocritical Care Society

Preface

Neurocritical care as a subspecialty has grown rapidly over the last two decades with the advent of newer monitoring, diagnostic, and therapeutic modalities in a variety for brain and spinal cord injury paradigms. The number of training programs and neurocritical care units has evolved over the last few years. The spectrum of diseases encompassed by the discipline is broad and includes traumatic brain injury, subarachnoid, intracerebral, and intraventricular hemorrhage, large hemispheric infarctions, status epilepticus, infections, and neuromuscular disorders such as Guillain-Barre syndrome and myasthenia gravis. Time is of the essence for rapid diagnoses and therapeutic interventions in many of these patients. The care provided to these patients is frequently multidisciplinary and includes emergency medical services personnel, emergency medicine physicians, neurologists, neurosurgeons, anesthesiologists, critical care physicians, and critical care nurses. Although the need for specialized care of this challenging subset of patients is clearly recognized, much is required for the education of first-line physicians and other health care providers in the importance of early recognition and timely therapeutic intervention in patients experiencing acute neurological deterioration.

The *Handbook of Neurocritical Care* should serve as a quick reference guide for those involved in the care of critically ill neurological and neurosurgical patients. It is not meant to substitute for a full-length text in the discipline. This handbook provides an algorithmic approach incorporating ancillary investigations to confirm clinical diagnosis and to provide appropriate management of acute neurological diseases for first-line health care providers. Tables and illustrations are provided for quick and easy bedside reference for residents and fellows-in-training. Staff in units other than neurology and neurosurgery who are involved in the management of neurologically ill patients will also find this book helpful.

In an attempt to present succinct information, contributing authors for the *Handbook of Neurocritical Care* are both trainees and faculty from our Johns Hopkins team. Key Points at the end of each chapter highlighting the essential elements should serve as a quick summary for the reader. We hope you find this handbook useful.

The editors are indebted to the contributors for their valuable contributions. Special thanks are due to Patricia M. Lamberti and Gloria A. McCoy for their efforts in coordinating the development of this book. We would also like to particularly express our thanks to the Johns Hopkins Clinician Scientist Program, the Dana Foundation, American Heart Association, National Stroke Association, American Academy of Neurology, American Epilepsy Society, and the National Institutes of Health extramural programs that have supported our investigative work and fellowship training program in neurocritical care over the years. Finally, we would like to take this opportunity to recognize the pioneering efforts of Daniel F. Hanley, Cecil O. Borel, Judith Ski Lower, and the unit nursing leadership who worked tirelessly to establish the program and maintain a collaborative specialty model of care at Johns Hopkins University School of Medicine that has lead to the growth of this discipline.

Anish Bhardwaj, MD,
Marek A. Mirski, MD, PhD,
John A. Ulatowski, MD, PhD, MBA

Contents

Contributors

AGNIESZKA A. ARDELT, MD, PhD • Fellow, Neurosciences Critical Care Division, Johns Hopkins University School of Medicine, Baltimore, MD

LAUREN BERKOW, MD • Director, Airway Services; Assistant Professor of Anesthesiology/Critical Care Medicine; Staff Attending, Johns Hopkins Hospital, Johns Hopkins University School of Medicine, Baltimore, MD

ANISH BHARDWAJ, MD • Associate Professor of Neurology, Anesthesiology/Critical Care Medicine and Neurological Surgery; Vice Chairman, Department of Neurology; Co-Director, Neurosciences Critical Care Division; Staff Attending, Neurosciences Critical Care Unit, Johns Hopkins Hospital, Johns Hopkins University School of Medicine, Baltimore, MD

CHERE M. CHASE, MD • Fellow, Neurosciences Critical Care Division, Johns Hopkins University School of Medicine, Baltimore, MD

CONNIE L. CHEN, MD • Fellow, Neurosciences Critical Care Division, Johns Hopkins University School of Medicine, Baltimore, MD

ROMERGRYKO G. GEOCADIN, MD • Assistant Professor of Neurology, Anesthesiology/Critical Care Medicine and Neurological Surgery; Director, Neurocritical Care Unit, Bayview Medical Center; Staff Attending, Neurosciences Critical Care Unit, Johns Hopkins Hospital and Bayview Medical Center, Johns Hopkins University School of Medicine, Baltimore, MD

MITZI K. HEMSTREET, MD, PhD • Western Pennsylvania Anesthesia Associates, Allegheny General Hospital, Pittsburgh, PA

GEOFFREY S. F. LING, MD, PhD • Professor and Vice Chairman, Department of Neurology; Director, Neurosciences Critical Care, Uniformed Services University of the Health Sciences, Bethesda, MD

MAREK A. MIRSKI, MD, PhD • Associate Professor of Anesthesiology/ Critical Care Medicine, Neurology and Neurological Surgery; Director, Neurosciences Critical Care Division; Chief, Neuroanesthesiology; Staff Attending, Neurosciences Critical Care Unit, Johns Hopkins Hospital and Bayview Medical Center, Johns Hopkins University School of Medicine, Baltimore, MD

ROBERT D. STEVENS, MD • Assistant Professor of Anesthesiology/Critical Care Medicine; Staff Attending, Neurosciences Critical Care Unit, Johns Hopkins Hospital and Bayview Medical Center; Johns Hopkins University School of Medicine, Baltimore, MD

MICHEL T. TORBEY, MD, MPH • Assistant Professor of Neurology and Anesthesiology/Critical Care Medicine; Director, Neurovascular Sonology, Neurosciences Critical Care Division; Staff Attending, Neurosciences Critical Care Unit, Johns Hopkins Hospital and Bayview Medical Center, Johns Hopkins University School of Medicine, Baltimore, MD

JOHN A. ULATOWSKI, MD, PhD, MBA • Professor of Anesthesiology/ Critical Care Medicine, Associate Professor of Neurology and Neurological Surgery; Chairman, Department of Anesthesiology/Critical Care Medicine; Staff Attending, Neurosciences Critical Care Unit, Johns Hopkins Hospital, Johns Hopkins University School of Medicine, Baltimore, MD

MICHAEL A. WILLIAMS, MD • Assistant Professor of Neurology and Neurological Surgery; Co-Chair, Ethics Committee; Core Faculty, Berman Bioethics Institute; Director, Adult Hydrocephalus Program, Johns Hopkins Hospital, Johns Hopkins University School of Medicine, Baltimore, MD

WENDY L. WRIGHT, MD • Fellow, Neurosciences Critical Care Division, Johns Hopkins University School of Medicine, Baltimore, MD

WENDY C. ZIAI, MD • Assistant Professor of Neurology and Anesthesiology/Critical Care Medicine; Director of Clinical Research, Neurosciences Critical Care Division; Staff Attending, Neurosciences Critical Care Unit, Johns Hopkins Hospital and Bayview Medical Center, Johns Hopkins University School of Medicine, Baltimore, MD

Value-Added eBook/PDA

This book is accompanied by a value-added CD-ROM that contains an eBook version of the volume you have just purchased. This eBook can be viewed on your computer, and you can synchronize it to your PDA for viewing on your handheld device. The eBook enables you to view this volume on only one computer and PDA. Once the eBook is installed on your computer, you cannot download, install, or e-mail it to another computer; it resides solely with the computer to which it is installed. The license provided is for only one computer. The eBook can only be read using Adobe® Reader® 6.0 software, which is available free from Adobe Systems Incorporated at www.Adobe.com. You may also view the eBook on your PDA using the Adobe® PDA Reader® software that is also available free from Adobe.com.

You must follow a simple procedure when you install the eBook/PDA that will require you to connect to the Humana Press website in order to receive your license. Please read and follow the instructions below:

1. Download and install Adobe® Reader® 6.0 software
   You can obtain a free copy of the Adobe® Reader® 6.0 software at www.adobe.com

   *Note: If you already have the Adobe® Reader® 6.0 software installed, you do not need to reinstall it.

2. Launch Adobe® Reader® 6.0 software
3. Install eBook: Insert your eBook CD into your CD-ROM drive
   PC: Click on the "Start" button, then click on "Run"

   At the prompt, type "d:\ebookinstall.pdf" and click "OK"

   *Note: If your CD-ROM drive letter is something other than d: change the above command accordingly.

   MAC: Double click on the "eBook CD" that you will see mounted on your desktop.

   Double click "ebookinstall.pdf"

4. Adobe® Reader® 6.0 software will open and you will receive the message
   "This document is protected by Adobe DRM" Click "OK"

   *Note: If you have not already activated the Adobe® Reader® 6.0 software, you will be prompted to do so. Simply follow the directions to activate and continue installation.

Your web browser will open and you will be taken to the Humana Press eBook registration page. Follow the instructions on that page to complete installation. You will need the serial number located on the sticker sealing the envelope containing the CD-ROM.

If you require assistance during the installation, or you would like more information regarding your eBook and PDA installation, please refer to the eBookManual.pdf located on your CD. If you need further assistance, contact Humana Press eBook Support by e-mail at ebooksupport@humanapr.com or by phone at 973-256-1699.

*Adobe and Reader are either registered trademarks or trademarks of Adobe Systems Incorporated in the United States and/or other countries.

1 Coma and Altered Consciousness

Wendy C. Ziai

Consciousness

♦ Active process often defined as the state of awareness of both self and the environment. Consciousness depends on two essential components:
  – **Arousal** Anatomic basis—ascending reticular activating system (RAS): Rostral pontine and mesencephalic tegmentum and midline and intralaminar thalamic nuclei
  – **Awareness** Requires cerebral cortex and its connections to the subcortical structures
    • **Cognition** Involves other components such as attention, sensation and perception, explicit memory, executive function, and motivation, and also depends on cerebral cortical activity

Disorders of Consciousness

♦ Caused by damage or suppression of the brainstem RAS or of both cerebral hemispheres
♦ Different states of altered consciousness can be defined, some of which have specific anatomical correlates
  – Coma
    • Sleep-like state of unresponsiveness with absence of awareness of self or environment and failure to respond to stimuli
    • Movements are pathologic or do not exist although degree of motor impairment is variable
    • The eyes do not open spontaneously or respond to stimulation. Sleep–wake cycles are absent
  – Stupor
    • State of reduced mental and physical activity in which patient can be roused only by repeated and vigorous stimuli. Patient lapses back into unresponsive state when the stimulus stops

From: *Current Clinical Neurology: Handbook of Neurocritical Care*
Edited by: A. Bhardwaj, M. A. Mirski, J. A. Ulatowski © Humana Press Inc., Totowa, NJ

- Verbal response is slow and incomplete or absent
- Motor responses are often restless and stereotyped
- Obtundation
  - State of mental dullness or blunting with increased sleeping time
  - Patient can be aroused to obey commands but maintains a reduced interest in the environment as well as slowed responses to stimulation
- Hypersomnia
  - Increase in sleeping time with normal sleep–wake cycles
  - Associated with sleep deprivation, metabolites of sedative drugs, acute hepatic or renal failure, or damage to brainstem/thalamic RAS regions
  - May be limited to states of excessive but normal sleep where patient can be roused readily when stimulated, even if only briefly
- Persistent Vegetative State
  - State of complete unawareness in which patient may open eyes spontaneously or respond to verbal stimuli without recognition of the environment
  - No localizing motor movements or ability to follow commands
  - This condition often follows a period of sleep-like coma and is associated with sleep–wake cycles as well as normal circulatory, brainstem, and respiratory function Diagnosis should not be made earlier than 1 mo after nontraumatic brain injury or 1 yr after traumatic brain insults
  - Nontraumatic vegetative states lasting >1 mo provide no chance of recovery beyond severe disability
  - Traumatic vegetative states lasting 1–6 mo offer a 25% chance of recovery to good or moderate disability
- Minimally Conscious State
  - A condition of severely altered consciousness in which minimal but definite behavioral evidence of self- or environmental awareness is demonstrated
  - Patients must have one or more of the following on a reproducible basis:
    □ Ability to follow simple commands
    □ Ability to signal yes/no responses regardless of accuracy
    □ Intelligible verbalization
    □ Nonreflexive movements in response to a stimulus or affective behavior

- Brain Death
  - State of irreversible loss of all brain and brainstem function, implying absence of consciousness, motor response to painful stimuli, and all brainstem reflexes including respiratory drive
- Locked-In Syndrome
  - State of selective de-efferentation of all four extremeties and lower cranial nerves, resulting in complete paralysis with inability to communicate by vocalization, but preservation of vertical eye movements and blinking because of sparing of oculomotor pathways in the midbrain
  - Typically caused by pontine infarction
  - Respiratory function is normal because of sparing of chemoreceptors in ventral medulla
  - Consciousness is preserved unless the RAS in the tegmentum is involved
  - Hearing is intact
- Akinetic Mutism
  - State of little or no awareness, immobility, and little or no vocalization that also occurs in certain chronic states of altered consciousness
  - Apparent absence of mental activity or spontaneous motor activity. Sleep–wake cycles are intact
  - Patient usually lies with the eyes closed but with periods of apparent wakefulness
  - Patient is incontinent and makes minimal motor movement to noxious stimuli
  - Many different lesions including large bifrontal lobe lesions, bihemispheric demyelination, and severe damage to the cerebral cortex
- Acute Confusional State
  - State of impaired attention, memory, and logical thinking in addition to incoherent conversation and susceptibility to distractions
  - Delerium is diagnosed if systemic manifestations (autonomic dysfunction) with fever, tachycardia, hypertension, and sweating are also present in combination with restlessness, agitation, and frequent hallucinations
  - These states usually do not cause stupor or coma, but they may precede metabolic stupor/coma and if untreated can lead to exhaustion and even death

Table1
Classification and Major Causes of Coma

Structural brain injury
    Hemisphere
        Unilateral (with displacement)
            Intraparenchymal hematoma
            Middle cerebral artery (MCA) occlusion with swelling
            Hemorrhagic contusion
            Cerebral abscess
            Brain tumor
        Bilateral
            Penetrating traumatic brain injury
            Multiple traumatic brain contusions
            Multiple cerebral cortical infarcts (vasculitis,
                coagulopathy, cardiac thrombus)
            Bilateral thalamic infarcts
            Lymphoma
            Encephalitis (viral, paraneoplastic)
            Gliomatosis
            Acute disseminated encephalomyelitis
            Anoxic–ischemic encephalopathy
            Cerebral edema
            Multiple brain metastases
            Acute hydrocephalus
            Leukoencephalopathy (chemotherapy or radiation)
    Brain stem
        Pontine hemorrhage
        Basilar artery occlusion
        Central ponine myelinolysis
        Brain stem hemorrhagic contusion
    Cerebellum (with displacement)
        Cerebellar infarct
        Cerebellar hematoma
        Cerebellar abscess
        Cerebellar tumor
Acute metabolic-endocrine derangement
        Hypoglycemia
        Hyperglycemia (nonketotic hyperosmolar)
        Hyponatremia
        Hypernatremia
        Addison's disease

(continued)

Table1 *(continued)*

Hypercalcemia
    Acute panhypopituitarism
    Acute uremia
    Hyperbilirubinemia
    Hypercapnia
Diffuse physiologic brain dysfunction
    Generalized tonic–clonic seizures
    Poisoning and illicit drug use
    Hypothermia
    Gas inhalation
    Basilar migraine
    Idiopathic recurrent stupor
Psychogenic unresponsiveness
    Acute (lethal) catatonia, malignant neuroleptic syndrome
    Hysterical coma
    Malingering

Adapted from EFM Wijdicks;2002:3–42.

- Acute delirium is frequent in intensive care unit patients, and is often associated with postoperative states, sensory deprivation, and drugs (intoxications and withdrawals)

Initial Evaluation and Management

♦ Monitor vital signs. Assume C-spine injury with trauma.
♦ Airway, Breathing, and Circulation
  – Establish an airway and deliver oxygen if signs of respiratory distress: shallow and irregular respirations, stertorous breathing, and cyanosis) are exhibited. Use head-tilt/chin-lift or jaw-thrust/head-tilt techniques to open airway. Place oropharyngeal airway (especially in patients who have had recent seizures)
  – Lateral decubitus position if not contraindicated by possible cervical spine trauma
  – Suction to prevent aspiration
  – Use mask ventilation followed by intubation and positive pressure ventilation if unable to protect airway and there is evidence of hypoxia or hypoventilation. Consider fiberoptic intubation if potential spinal cord injury
  – If severe upper airway obstruction or oropharyngeal bleeding makes intubation impossible, perform needle cricothyroidotomy:

14-gage needle inserted through cricothyroid membrane followed by insertion of a cannula. Jet insufflation of airway can be performed temporarily, followed by a surgical cricothyroidotomy. Monitor oxygenation with a pulse oximter (O_2 saturation should exceed 90%)
– *Caution:* elevation of intracranial pressure (ICP) may occur with hypoventilation and improper preparation for rapid sequence laryngoscopy and intubation. Except in rare circumstances use general anesthesia to blunt ICP rise to intubation
– Arterial blood gases: aim for PaO_2 >100 mmHg and low normal $PaCO_2$ (35–40 mmHg)
– Evaluate blood pressure and pulse rate. **Hypotension** has large differential in the comatose patient and is rarely caused by the intracranial injury unless patient is already brain dead or has a high spinal cord injury. Consider:
  • Myocardial infarction
  • Pulmonary embolism
  • Sepsis
  • Toxic effects of ingestions
  • Major abdominal or chest trauma
– Management should include the following: fluid resuscitation with isotonic saline (and blood if necessary) followed by vasopressors if inadequate response to fluids alone
– **Hypertension** is common in patients with acute brain injury, either as a result of increased sympathetic tone, certain drug ingestions (amphetamines, cocaine), or as part of a Cushing response in patients with increased ICP and herniation syndromes. The management of acute hypertension depends on the presumed etiology, chronicity, and risk for cerebral edema and cerebral ischemia. In general patients with intracerebral hemorrhages (ICHs) should have systolic blood pressure controlled to <160 mmHg whereas patients with ischemic lesions may require substantially higher cerebral perfusion pressures (CPP) to maintain adequate cerebral blood flow (CBF). β-Blockers such as labetolol, starting at 10–20 mg IV at 10 min intervals are the usual first line agent as a result of their minimal effect on cerebral hemodynamics
– Obtain intravenous access
– Assess body temperature. Core temperature below 34°C defines **hypothermia**. Nonenvironmental hypothermia may be caused by endocrine disorders (hypopituitarism, hypothyroidism), drugs (alcohol, barbiturates, general anesthetics), Wernicke's encephalopathy and, rarely, central disorders involving the dien-

cephalon. At body temperatures below 27°C brainstem reflexes are lost. Treatment of hypothermia includes warming blankets (32–35°C), warmed intravenous infusions (30–32°C), and peritoneal lavage with heated dialysate (<30°C). **Hyperthermia** may be caused by systemic sepsis, thyrotoxic crisis, heat stroke, drug toxicity, and malignant hyperthermia. Central hyperpyrexia is unusual, but can occur with subarachnoid hemorrhage, or hypothalamic lesions. Patients should be cooled to at least normothermia using cooling blankets, ice packs or alcohol baths, with addition of iced gastric lavage or cold saline infusions if necessary
– Electrocardiogram. Cardiac arrhythmias are frequently seen in brain-injured patients. **Tachycardia** may result from hypovolemia, fever, drugs or toxins, and increased sympathetic tone associated with intracranial injury. **Bradycardia** may reflect raised ICP, spinal cord injury or drug effect. Narrowing of the QRS interval may be an indication of severity of tricyclic antidepressant overdose Transient signs of **myocardial ischemia** may occur with intracranial hemorrhage, stroke, or traumatic brain injury and must be differentiated from primary cardiac injury by serial evaluation of cardiac enzymes and troponin levels, and echocardiography. **Malignant cardiac arrhythmias** (ventricular fibrillation, ventricular tachycardia) may occur with amphetamine overdose

Initial Diagnostic Workup and Medical Management

♦ Draw blood samples—screening laboratory analysis for readily correctable conditions (*see* Table 2)
♦ Thiamine: 100 mg IV, followed by 25 g of glucose IV (50 mL of a 50% solution). Do not delay potentially life-saving treatment of **hypoglycemia**, although hyperglycemia is injurious to neurons Thiamine is administered prior to glucose to avoid precipitation of **Wernicke's encephalopathy** in malnourished or alcoholic patients
♦ Naloxone (0.4–2 mg IV q3 min, or infusion 0.8 mg/kg/h) should be given if **narcotic overdose** is a possibility. Potential serious side effects include aspiration pneumonitis as a result of rapid arousal, florid withdrawal syndrome
♦ Flumazenil (0.2 mg/min up to 1 mg IV) can be given for **benzodiazepine overdose**. Flumazenil can precipitate cardiac arrhythmias as well as the same side effects as naloxone. It is contraindicated for possible ingestion of tricyclic antidepressants, or in patients with active seizures as a result of lowered seizure threshold and possibility of inducing status epilepticus

Table 2
Initial Examination of a Comatose Patient

Physical examination

1. ABC: Initial resuscitation
2. Respiration: Upper/lower airway dysfunction
3. Overall level of consciousness
4. Cranial nerve exam (looking for focal lesion)
   - Eye movements
   - Pupillary responses
   - Oculocephalic/vestibuloocular reflex
   - Corneal, cough, and gag reflexes
5. Motor exam (looking for asymmetry)
   - Resting posture
   - Spontaneous motor activity
   - Response to stimulation
6. Systemic exam: temperature, fundoscopic, ears, nose, and throat, integument, cardiac/vascular, abdomen.
7. Laboratory studies:
   - Glucose: hypoglycemia, nonketotic hyperglycemia, diabetic
   - Ketoacidosis
   - Complete blood count: sepsis
   - Urinalysis: urosepsis
   - Electrolytes: hyponatremia, hypernatremia
   - Calcium: hypercalcemia, hypocalcemia
   - Magnesium: hypermagnesemia
   - Liver function tests: hyperbilirubinemia, hyperammonemia
   - Renal function tests: acute uremia
   - Thyroid function tests: acute hypothyroidism
   - Urine toxicology screen: intoxication
   - Arterial blood gas analysis: hypoxia, hypercapnia
   - Lactate: lactic acidosis
8. Other investigations

Investigation	Indication
Computed tomography (CT) scan brain	Almost any unconscious patient especially with focal signs
Lumbar puncture	Suspected meningitis, encephalitis, or occult subarachnoid hemorrhage
Angiogram	Suspected basilar artery thrombosis
Electroechocardiogram (EEG)	Suspected nonconvulsive status epilepticus and monitoring of seizing patient during treatment.
Magnetic resonance imaging (MRI)/MRV	Suspected cerebral venous sinus thrombosis, basilar artery thromosis, cerebellar or brainstem infarction not well visualized on CT Adjunctive test for herpes simplex encephalitis

Note: Focal findings imply mass lesions and hasten need for imaging studies.

♦ **Drug ingestion** is treated with activated charcoal (60–100 g) and normal saline lavage in patients who have a protected airway. Caustic substances should not be lavaged. Hemodialysis may be required to clear toxins such as acetaminophen, amitryptiline, lithium, and salicylates

♦ Other acute metabolic derangements are treated as follows:

  – **Hyponatremia** If severe (serum sodium <125 meq/L) should be treated with hypertonic saline (2 or 3% maintenance or bolus infusions) with careful monitoring of serum sodium every 4–6 h. Over rapid correction of sodium has been associated with central pontine myelinolysis. Lesser degrees of hyponatremia can be managed with sodium chloride tablets (2 g q6h PO) and free water restriction

  – **Hypercalcemia** Saline rehydration infusion of several liters as tolerated followed by intravenous bisphosphonate pamidronate (60 mg over 24 h)

♦ **Systemic examination and history** Interview relatives or friends of patient early on to establish circumstances in which patient was found, onset and progression of loss of consciousness, preexisting conditions, and drug or alcohol history. General medical evaluation may quickly reveal acute diagnoses as well as chronic conditions (*see* Table 3)

Neurologic Examination

♦ Four major components: level of consciousness, cranial nerve examination, motor examination, and respiratory patterns

♦ **Glasgow Coma Scale** (GCS): standard scoring system for comatose patients (*see* Table 4). Designed for initial evaluation of head trauma patients. Reliable for predicting outcome after head trauma. Reproducible scale easily applied by medical and nursing staff. Limitations include:

  – Motor responses may be only reliable test in ventilated patient or patient with significant orbital swelling

  – Does not assess asymmetry and many other important neurologic functions

  – Mid-range scores (6–12) can occur with many different combinations of the three components which do not reflect the same degree of unconsciousness

  – Higher scores (10–15) do not predict significant differences in outcome

Table 3
Systemic Signs in Patients With Altered Consciousness

Physical signs	Potential significance
Head/ENT:	
Battle sign, racoon's eyes, otorrhea, rhinorhea	Basal skull fracture
Meningismus	Meningitis, subarachnoid hemorrhage (SAH)
Eyelid edema	Myedema coma, cavernous sinus thrombosis
Mucous membranes	Cyanosis or carbon monoxide intoxication
Fundoscopy:	
Papilledema	Increased ICP, hypertensive encephalopathy, acute asphyxia
Retinal hemorrhage, subhyaloid hemorrhage, Tersons Syndrome: hemorrhage within vitreous humor	Trauma, SAH
Retinopathy	Hypertension, diabetes
Skin	
Dry skin	Anticholinergic/barbiturate poisoning
Wet skin	Cholinergic poisoning, hypoglycemia, sympathomimetic agents, sympathetic storm, thyroid storm
Purpura	Meningococcal meningitis, disseminated intravascular coagulation (DIC), vasculitis, thrombocytopenic purpura
Ecchymosis/petichiae	Trauma, steroids, liver disease, anticoagulants, DIC, ribothymidine 5'-triphosphate TTP
Rash, purpura, petichiae	Meningitis, DIC, sepsis, endocarditis
Maculopapular rash	Viral meningoencephalitis, endocariditis, fungal infection
Vesicular rash	Herpes simplex virus or varicella infection
Bullae, blisters	Barbiturate overdose
Hyperpigmentation	Addison's disease, porphyria, malignant melanoma, chemotherapy

(continued)

Table 3 *(continued)*

Physical signs	Potential significance
Peculiar odors on the breath:	
Musty	Uremia
Fruity	Ketoacidosis
Fishy	Acute hepatic failure
Cardiopulmonary	
Cardiac murmurs	Infective endocarditis
Arrhythmias	Cardiac emboli
Gastrointestinal	
Jaundice	Hepatic encephalopathy
Acute abdomen (ruptured abdominal viscus or aneurysm)	Sepsis, continued dissection or bleeding

Table 4
Glasgow Coma Scale

Eye opening	4	Spontaneous
	3	To speech
	2	To pain
	1	None
Motor response	6	Obeys command
	5	Localizes pain
	4	Withdrawal
	3	Flexion posturing
	2	Extensor posturing
	1	None
Verbal response	5	Oriented
	4	Confused speech
	3	Inappropriate words
	2	Incomprehensible sounds
	1	None

– Requires regular and serial observations to be effective, but has insufficient sensitivity to detect subtle changes in level of consciousness (LOC), that may have significance in trauma patients and those with mass lesions

Table 5
States of Altered Level of Consciousness

Feature	Coma	PVS	Brain death	Locked-In syndrome	Akinetic mutism	Dementia
Self-awareness	Absent	Absent	Absent	Present	Present	Variable
Sleep–wake cycles	Absent	Present	Absent	Present	Present	Present
Motor function	None purposeful	None purposeful	None purposeful	Limited to vertical eye movements Quadriplegia + bulbar palsies	Extreme paucity of movement	Variable
Respiratory function	Variable	Intact	Absent	Intact	Intact	Intact
Suffering	No	No	No	Yes	Yes	Variable
EEG	Variable; depends on severity	Polymorphic theta and delta; slow alpha	Electro-cerebral silence	Usually normal	Non-specific slowing	Usually slowing
Cerebral metabolism	<50%	<50%	Absent	Variable	Variable	Variable
Prognosis	Usually known in 2 wk	Traumatic: 25% chance of good outcome or moderate disability at 6 mo; Nontraumatic: severe disability or death	None	Recovery unlikely; prolonged survival possible; remain quadriplegic	Recovery unlikely; depends on cause	Recovery unlikely

♦ Level of Consciousness
 – Establish level of unresponsiveness; differentiate unconscious-ness from psychogenic coma or paralysis with intact awareness (locked-in syndrome) (*see* Table 5)
 – Observe for spontaneous motor movement, eye movements, and body position.
 – Positions of comfort (e.g., crossing the legs, yawning) generally indicate less impairment
 – Use verbal stimuli and simple commands prior to noxious stimulation
♦ Cranial Nerve Examination
 –Eye movements

Table 6
Eye Movements and Position

Eye position/movement	*Anatomical localization*
Horizontal conjugate deviation to side of lesion (away from side of paralysis)	Hemisphere (involving frontal eye fields)
Horizontal conjugate deviation opposite side of lesion (ipsilateral to paralyzed side)	Horizontal gaze center in pons; can occur with thalamic injury ("wrong way eyes") or central brain herniation
Disconjugate gaze	Cranial nerve palsy or damage to brainstem tegmentum
Skew deviation	Lesion in brainstem or cerebellum involving vertical vestibulo-ocular pathways (typically vascular lesions of pons or lateral medulla)
Ocular bobbing	Severe central pontine injury
Ocular dipping/reverse ocular bobbing	Severe metabolic or structural damage involving midbrain/diencephalic region
Ping pong gaze (horizontal conjugate eye deviation alternating every few seconds)	Bilateral cerebral or upper brainstem damage, or metabolic dysfunction
Tonic downward deviation of gaze	Thalamus or dorsal midbrain: medial thalamic hemorrhage, acute obstructive hydrocephalus, severe metabolic or hypoxic encephalopathy, massive subarachnoid hemorrhage
Tonic upward deviation of gaze	Bilateral hemispheric damage (cardiac arrest, hypotension) with relative sparing of brainstem
Brief upward gaze spasm (oculogyric crisis)	Neuroleptic drugs, cyclosporine toxicity
Periodic alternating gaze	Hepatic encephalopathy, bihemispheric midbrain or vermis lesions
Roving eye movements	Nonlocalizing; disappear with brainstem injury
Convergence nystagmus	Midbrain lesion

- Eye opening is not synonymous with awareness (as in the persistent vegetative state) and comatose patients may have the eyes open
- Spontaneous eye movements and their pattern as well as eye position and deviation should be noted (*see* Table 6)

Table 7
Oculocephalic and Vestibulo-Ocular Responses

Site of lesion	Response description
None; normal awake patient, or psychogenic unresponsiveness	OCR: inconsistent or fixation on target VOR (CWC): nystagmus (fast component away from irrigated ear), intense nausea, vertigo, vomiting
Diffuse or bilateral hemisphere dysfunction with intact brainstem	OCR: contralateral conjugate eye deviation VOR (CWC): tonic conjugate deviation of both eyes toward irrigated ear; slow return to midline; no nystagmus
Low brainstem lesion	OCR: None VOR (CWC): no response; no nystagmus
Bilateral medial longitudinal fasciculus injury	OCR: Appropriate eye deviates laterally away from direction of head turning; eye which would deviate medially deviates only to midline. VOR (CWC): ipsilateral eye deviates laterally toward irrigated ear; contralateral eye deviates only to midline; no nystagmus

Abbr: OCR, oculocephalic reflex; VOR, vestibulo-ocluar reflex; CWC, cold water calorics

- Spontaneous nystagmus may be seen in diffuse brain injury or with epilepsy
- Intermittent horizontal gaze preference, nystagmoid eye movements, and eyelid myoclonus indicate possible seizures
- The horizontal gaze center and medial longitudinal fasciculus are tested with the oculocephalic (absence of cervical spine trauma) and vestibulo-ocular reflexes (cold water calorics). Damage to the internuclear pathways will allow only abduction of the eye ipsilateral to cold water irrigation. Nystagmus to the opposite side implies intact brainstem function and cortical correction. Vertical eye movements can be tested using these

Table 8
Pupillary Size and Reaction to Light

Pupillary abnormality	Neuroanatomical significance
Sudden unilateral fixed dilated pupil	Ipsilateral uncal herniation causing compression of the third nerve and/or nucleus; posterior communicating artery aneurysm (classically) or other compressive lesion along the course of the oculomotor nerve.
Unilateral miosis	Horner's syndrome: sympathetic denervation
Bilateral fixed dilated pupils	Some massive overdoses (carbamazepine, tricyclic antidepressants, amphetamines); antibiotic-induced paralysis; large doses of atropine or dopamine, but with preserved pupillary reaction to light
Mid-position fixed pupils	Extensive brainstem destruction; end-stage herniation, brain death
Bilateral miosis (pupillary light reflex usually preserved)	High doses of narcotics, pontine injury (hemorrhage), nonketotic hyperglycemia, organophosphates or miotic eye drops

manoeuvers as well and may help identify infarctions restricted to the thalamus or rostral midbrain
- Visual fields, pupillary size, and reaction to light
  • Visual fields can be tested by presence of blink reflex to threat on moving the hand suddenly toward the patient's eye from all quadrants
  • Pupillary size and reaction to light assess upper brainstem function and some drug effects (*see* Table 8). Anisocoria is defined as difference in pupil diameter of >1 mm. Abnormal pupillary shapes include oval pupils
  • The pupillary light reflex is usually spared by toxic and metabolic causes of coma although pupillary size may be affected symmetrically.

Table 9
Motor Responses in Comatose Patients

Common motor responses	*Anatomic site of lesion*
Flexion in an upper extremity	Incomplete contralateral cerebral lesion
Extension in an upper extremity	Deep cerebral or brainstem lesions
Triple flexion in lower extremity	Nonlocalizing spinal reflex
Decorticate posturing (Flexion and adduction of arms and wrists; extension of lower extremities)	Damage to thalamus or cerebral hemispheres with structures below the diencephalon remaining intact. Subcortical pathways released from higher control centers.
Decerebrate posturing (Adduction, extension, pronation of arms and wrists; extension of lower extremities)	Deep bilateral cerebral hemisphere lesions, bilateral damage to midbrain and upper pons (above vestibular nuclei), and severe metabolic disorders such as anoxia.
Flaccid; absent response to painful stimulus	Damage to the lower medulla or widespread central or peripheral nervous system damage.

- Cranial Nerves 5 and 7
  • The fifth and seventh cranial nerves are tested with the corneal reflex. The response to stimulating the inside of the nostrils is also useful but should be avoided in patients with potential cribriform plate fractures
  • Presence of facial palsy can be assessed by asymmetry of grimace response to central pain. Asymmetry of the lower face only (sparing the frontalis muscle) indicates a central lesion versus a peripheral facial palsy (both upper and lower facial muscles affected)
- Cranial Nerves 9 and 10
  • The ninth and tenth cranial nerves should be tested by tracheal suctioning (unless spontaneous coughing occurs) or other direct stimulation of the posterior pharynx. Sedative drugs (narcotics and neuromuscular blocking agents used for intubation) may suppress this response
♦ Motor Responses
  - Observe resting posture, spontaneous motor activity, and response to stimulation. Common involuntary movements include

Table 10
Classical Respiratory Patterns in Coma

Respiratory pattern	Anatomic localization/etiology
Cheyne–Stokes Respirations (hyperpnea regularly alternating with apnea)	Bilateral cerebral dysfunction Increased ICP Decreased cardiac output
Short-cycle Cheyne–Stokes breathing	ICH
Biot's breathing (irregular Cheyne–Stokes)	Incomplete lower brainstem failure
Central neurogenic hyperventilation (with respiratory alkalosis)	Damage to rostral brainstem tegmentum paramedian pontine reticular formation. May be caused by stimulation of afferent peripheral reflexes in lung and chest wall by pulmonary congestion.
Apneusis (deep breathing; brief end-inspiratory pauses alternating with end-expiratory pauses)	Respiratory control areas in mid-caudal pons (pontine infarction); rarely seen with transtentorial herniation
Ataxic breathing (irregular, deep and shallow breaths)	Reticular formation of dorsomedial medulla down to obex; rapid medullary compression

seizures, myoclonus (seen in anoxic encephalopathy and other metabolic comas) and certain tremors associated with acute confusional states as a result of toxic or metabolic etiologies. Motor responses to painful stimuli may be reflexive, purposeful, or absent and have some localizing value (*see* Table 9)

– Apply stimulus to the inner aspect of the upper arm and leg as opposed to peripheral sites (nail bed) that may be more difficult to interpret as withdrawal vs brainstem spinal reflex

◆ Respiratory Patterns in Coma

– Caused by reduced level of consciousness, or injury to brainstem respiratory centers.

– Upper airway dysfunction: Associated with decreased tone and strength of oropharynx and tongue or edema. Decreased PaO_2 and increased $PaCO_2$

– Lower airway dysfunction: results from intercostal muscle weakness or diaphragmatic paralysis. Ventilatory insufficiency: reduced vital capacity and increased $PaCO_2$

– Localizing value of classical breathing patterns: often unreliable because of overlapping metabolic and neurogenic influences on breathing

Key Points

♦ Cardiopulmonary stabilization to prevent secondary brain injury in comatose patients; most importantly early endotracheal intubation, and maintaining cerebral perfusion

♦ Serial examinations should be performed to detect early deterioration

♦ Avoid both hypovolemia and overhydration in comatose patients. The goal is to achieve a euvolemic state

♦ Look for readily correctable causes (hypoxia, hypoglycemia) and focal signs on examination (mass lesions)

♦ Return to the history when available to establish a time course

Suggested Reading

Cordova S and Lee R. Fixed dilated pupils in the ICU: another recoverable cause. *Anaesth Intensive Care* 2000;2891–2893.

Giacino JT and Kalmar K. The vegetative and minimally conscious states: a comparison of clinical features and functional outcome. *J Head Trauma Rehabil* 1997;12:36–51.

Gueye PN, Hoffman JR, Taboulet P, et al. Empiric use of flumazenil in comatose patients: limited applicability of criteria to define low risk. *Ann Emerg Med* 1996;27:730.

Hoffman JR, Schriger DL, Luo JS. The empiric use of naloxone in patients with altered mental status: a reappraisal. *Ann Emerg Med* 1996;20:246.

Mercer WN, Childs NL. Coma, vegetative state, and the minimally conscious state: diagnosis and management. *The Neurologist* 1999;5: 186–193.

The Multi-Society Task Force on PVS. Medical aspects of the persistent vegetative state. *N Engl J Med*1994;330:1499–1508, 1572–1579.

Plum F and Posner JB. The pathologic physiology of signs and symptoms of coma, in: *The Diagnosis of Stupor and Coma,* 3rd edition. Philadelphia: F.A. Davis Company;1982:1–86.

Wijdicks EFM. Altered arousal and coma, in: *Neurologic Catastrophes in the Emergency Room* Boston: Butterworth-Heinemann;2000:3–42.

Wijdicks EFM. Coma and other states of altered awareness, in: *Neurologic Complications of Critical Illness,* 2nd edition. New York: Oxford University Press; 2000:3–27.

2   Encephalopathy

Wendy L. Wright

Encephalopathy and Delirium

♦ Encephalopathy is an acute confusional state that is accompanied by an alteration in the level of consciousness (drowsiness, stupor, or coma)
- The term often used interchangeably with delirium

♦ Delirium is an acute, fluctuating state of confusion resulting from diffuse or multifocal cerebral dysfunction
- Delirium is characterized by impaired attention, concentration, orientation, and memory, fluctuations of consciousness, disordered thinking, hallucinations, incoherent speech, and agitation
- "Loud" delirium: hallucinations and psychomotor agitation
- "Quiet" delirium: decreased mental acuity and inattention. This is less easily recognized than "loud" delerium but probably equally dangerous. Mostcommon form in the elderly

♦ Avoid the notion of "intensive care unit (ICU) psychosis"; implies that encephalopathy is a consequence of the ICU stay and promotes complacency that may slow the search for all reversible precipitants
- Encephalopathy in the ICU patient is a reflection of underlying illness or fatigue, *NOT* a result of being in the ICU

♦ "Sundowning" is often used to describe a delerium that develops in an elderly (usually demented) patient at night with disturbed sleep–wake cycle; again, promotes complacency, so avoid

♦ Impact of encephalopathy: increased length of ICU stay, increased mortality, prolonged mechanical ventilation, and increased risk of self-injury (e.g., self-extubation, pulling supporting catheters)

From: *Current Clinical Neurology: Handbook of Neurocritical Care*
Edited by: A. Bhardwaj, M. A. Mirski, J. A. Ulatowski © Humana Press Inc., Totowa, NJ

Risk Factors

♦ Patients in an ICU are at high risk for encephalopathy because of:
  − Multisystem illnesses and comorbidities
  − Use of psychoactive medications
  − Advanced age
  − Malnutrition

Evaluation

♦ ABCs: assess adequacy of airway, breathing, and circulation
  − Vital signs: look for tachycardia, hypotension, and hypoxemia
  − Arterial blood gas (ABG): look for failure of oxygenation or ventilation
♦ History
♦ Physical examination
♦ Labs
  − Glucose
  − Toxicology screen
  − Urinalysis
    • Rule out infection
    • Urine porphobilinogens in selected cases when porphyria is suspected
  − Complete blood count (CBC)
  − Electrolytes (including Ca^{++}, Mg^{++})
  − Liver function tests, serum ammonia
  − Blood cultures
  − Thyroid function tests
♦ Diagnostic studies
  − Chest x-ray
  − Head computed tomography (CT)
  − Lumbar puncture (LP)
  − Electroencephalogram (EEG)
♦ Avoid sedation

Delirium Scales

♦ Need a monitoring and assessment device
♦ Many require a verbally responsive patient
♦ Intensive Care Delirium Screening checklist developed recently
  − Based on the presence of eight items
    • Altered level of consciousness
    • Inattention
    • Disorientation

- Hallucination or delusions
- Psychomotor agitation or retardation
- Inappropriate mood or speech
- Sleep–wake cycle disturbance
- Symptom fluctuation
  - A score of four items on this scale has 99% sensitivity and 64% specificity when used to screen for delirium
♦ Confusion Assessment Method (CAM)-ICU
  - Has four features, the evaluation of which can be adapted if the patient is mechanically ventilated. Delirium is present if the patient has both features 1 and 2, and either feature 3 or 4
    1. An acute onset of mental status changes or fluctuating course
    2. Inattention
    3. Disorganized thinking
    4. An altered level of consciousness

Differentiating Features of Encephalopathy, Delirium, and Dementia

♦ Dementia is a progressive disease involving disturbances in multiple spheres of cognition and not usually associated with a decreased level of consciousness early on
♦ Demented patients are more susceptible to developing encephalopathy

Treatment

♦ Focus on determining and treating underlying cause
  - Rapidly reversible causes: treatment
    - Wernicke's encephalopathy: thiamine, glucose
    - Opiate induced: Naloxone
    - Benzodiazepine induced: Flumazenil
  - Modification of environmental factors
    - Allow uninterrupted sleep as often as possible
    - Room with a window or a well-lit room
    - Close observation with frequent redirection and reorientation
♦ Symptomatic Treatment
  - May be considered when available and not contraindicated
  - Define goals of treatment (i.e., reduce risk of self-injury, reduce tachycardia, patient comfort)
  - Haldol: PO/IV/IM in small doses, titrated for effect
    - Risk of extrapyramidal side effects and paradoxical agitation
    - Can take up to 10 min to work

- Can worsen delirium in alcohol withdrawal and cocaine-induced encephalopathy. Benzodiazepines are the treatment of choice in these cases
  - Sedatives should be avoided if possible
  - Midazolam can be used if the patient is at risk of injuring self but repeated doses should be avoided
  - If restraints are used for patient safety they should be adjusted and checked periodically to prevent excessive constriction.

Causes and Management of Specific Causes of Encephalopathy

◆ Mild systemic illness commonly produces encephalopathy in elderly or demented patients, especially when combined with new medications, fever, or sleep deprivation

◆ In the neurocritical care unit causes of altered mentation may be neurologic. Toxic and metabolic causes, however, should not be overlooked and often play a significant role in the neurocritical care setting

◆ Toxic
  - Medications commonly used in the ICU
    - Opiates as analgesics
    - MSO_4, fentanyl, meperidine as epidural—rare cause of systemic toxicity
    - Benzodiazepines
    - Propofol
    - Steroids
  - Only in 5% of patients. Those who develop delirium often have an underlying affective or psychotic disorder
    - Acetylsalicylic acid
  - Neuroleptic malignant syndrome (*see* Chapter 4)
    - Encephalopathy, rigidity, hyperthermia, tachycardia, and hypertension are caused by neuroleptic medications such as haloperidol
    - Potentially fatal but can be treated with bromocriptine in mild cases, dantrolene in more severe cases
  - Industrial
    - Organophosphates
      □ Symptoms: bradycardia, hypotension, miosis, increased lacrimation, nausea and/or vomiting, diarrhea, encephalopathy, seizures, and coma
      □ Treatment: atropine, benzodiazepines, and phenytoin for seizures

- Carbon monoxide
  - ☐ Symptoms: Encephalopathy, dizziness, headache, tachycardia, ataxia, syncope and seizures
  - ☐ Treatment: 100% oxygen or hyperbaric oxygen
- Carbon disulfide
- Organic solvents
- Bromide
- Methyl chloride
- Heavy metals
  - ☐ Lead
  - ☐ Arsenic
  - ☐ Mercury
  - ☐ Bismuth
  - ☐ Thallium
  - ☐ Tin
- Environmental toxins
  - ☐ Plants and mushrooms
  - ☐ Venom (e.g., snakes, insects, fish)
- Inhalants
  - ☐ Gasoline
  - ☐ Glue
  - ☐ Ether
  - ☐ Nitrous oxide
  - ☐ Nitrates
- Illicit drugs
  - ☐ Cocaine
  - ☐ Heroin
  - ☐ Benzodiazepines
  - ☐ Lysergic Acid Diethylamide (LSD)
  - ☐ Phencyclidine (PCP)
- Withdrawal syndromes
  - ☐ Alcohol
    - ◊ Mild: Tremors, irritability, anorexia and nausea
      - o Symptoms usually appear within a few hours after reduction or cessation of alcohol intake, and tend to resolve within 48 h
      - o Symptoms may include dysphoria, insomnia, diaphoresis, impaired attention and concentration, tremors, and seizures
      - o Tend to occur 1–10 d after cessation of benzdiazepines, may last several days to weeks

◊ Severe: "delirium tremens"—carries significant mortality
 o Tremulousness, hallucinations, agitation, confusion, disorientation, and autonomic hyperactivity (fever, tachycardia, and diaphoresis) typically occur 72–96 h after cessation of drinking
 o Symptoms generally resolve within 3–5 d.
◊ Alcohol withdrawal seizures: typically one or a few brief generalized convulsions
 o Occur 12–48 h after cessation of alcohol intake
 o Antiepileptic drugs are not indicated for typical alcohol withdrawal seizures
 o Other causes for seizures must be excluded
◊ Secondary derangements: patients with alcohol withdrawal are susceptible to hypomagnesemia, hypokalemia, hypoglycemia, and fluid losses, mostly as a result of fever, diaphoresis, and vomiting
◊ If hypoglycemia is present, thiamine should be administered before glucose to prevent precipitation of Wernicke's encephalopathy
◊ Treatment
 o Chlordiazepoxide: 100 mg iv or PO q2–6 h as needed; Maximum dose: 500 mg in the first 24-h period. The initial 24-h dose can be administered again over the next 24 h, then the dosage can be reduced by 25–50mg per day each day thereafter
 o Lorazepam or other longer lasting benzodiazepines may facilitate smoother symptomatic control. Can be given 1–2 mg PO or IV q6–8 h as needed
 o Oxazepam 15–30 mg PO, q6–8 h as needed can be given to patients with hepatic failure, as it is excreted by the kidneys
 o Effective use of propofol drip has been reported.
 o Maintenance of fluid and electrolyte balance is important
 o Haloperidol should be avoided as it may cause paradoxical agitation
□ Nicotine withdrawal
◊ Signs and symptoms include bradycardia, depressed mood, anxiety, irritability, slowed cognition, sleep disruption, difficulty concentrating, increased appetite, and impatience

◊ Nicotine craving is most prominent within the first three days, and irritability, anxiety, and disturbed sleep peak at about 1 wk

◊ Treatment: 21 mg transdermal nicotine patch—anecdotal use in neurocritical care setting have not shown serious side effects

♦ Metabolic
  – Fluid disturbances
    • Dehydration: diabetes insipidus (DI), inadequate fluid administration
    • Water intoxication: psychogenic polydipsia, iatrogenic
  – Electrolyte disturbances
    • Hyponatremia
      □ Causes: edematous states (CHF, nephritic syndrome, cirrhosis), endocrine dysfunction (hypothyroidism, adrenal insufficiency), iatrogenic (postoperative fluid overload, medication-induced, hypotonic fluid administration), SIADH, "cerebral salt wasting"
        ◊ Post-op patients are at relatively high risk owing to stress, nausea, volume contraction, and medications
        ◊ SIADH is a major cause in patients with CNS disease (brain abscess or infection, brain tumor, head trauma, etc.)
          ○ Treatment is by fluid restriction, unless the patient has vasospasm following subaracnoid hemorrhage, then hypertonic saline administration may be required
        ◊ Centrally mediated renal sodium wasting (cerebral salt wasting)—existence of this syndrome is controversial
      □ Results in cellular swelling and brain edema
      □ Symptoms: weakness, confusion, disorientation, seizures, and coma
        ◊ Rapidity of development is an important determinant of symptoms
      □ Treatment
        ◊ Can be conservative if hyponatremia developed gradually (also, often less symptomatic)
        ◊ Balance risk of damage from hyponatremia vs risk of damage from central pontine myelinolysis
    • Hypernatremia
      □ Causes: extrarenal (insensible losses owing to fever, burns, mechanical ventilation, diarrhea, and sweat), renal

(osmotic diuresis, central DI, nephrogenic DI), iatrogenic
(hypertonic saline administration, medications)

◊ Typically will not develop if thirst mechanisms are
intact and if there is unrestricted access and ability to
drink water

□ Hyperosmolar state causes brain cells to shrink—brain
equilibrates to these in several hours, therefore these states
should be corrected slowly

□ Symptoms: agitation, seizures, lethargy, coma, and
seizures; intracranial bleeding can develop as the shrinking
brain pulls away from the meninges and bridging veins tear

– Glucose
  • Hypoglycemia

    □ Confusion, seizures, stupor, coma, and occasionally
    hemiparesis or other focal neurologic findings

    □ Typically caused by accidental or deliberate overdoses of
    insulin or antidiabetic agents, insulin-secreting islet cell
    tumors or retroperitoneal sarcoma, protracted ethanol intoxi-
    cation (in rare cases)

    □ Initial symptoms consist of nervousness, hunger, tachy-
    cardia, palpitations, anxiety, sweating, and tremor

      ◊ Frequently recognized by the patient and respond
      quickly to oral or parenteral glucose

    □ If the syndrome progresses, patients develop increasing
    confusion, drowsiness, motor restlessness, myoclonic twitch-
    ing, and seizures

  • Hyperglycemia

    □ Ketotic or non-ketotic

    □ May lead to encephalopathy or coma

– Calcium: hypocalcemia, hypercalcemia
– Magnesium: hypomagnesemia, hypermagnesemia
– Respiratory
  • Hypoxia
  • Hypercapnia

    □ Caused by underlying pulmonary disease or narcotic
    administration

    □ CO_2 retention can cause headache, papilledema, and
    altered levels of consciousness

    □ EEG frequently shows slowing in the theta and delta ranges

    □ Hypercapnia usually does not cause prolonged coma or
    irreversible brain damage

- □ Treatment
  - ◊ Intermittent positive pressure ventilation
  - ◊ Oxygen can be dangerous because it may blunt the respiratory drive but should be administered to raise arterial oxygen tension to between 50 and 55 mmHg
- • Pulmonary embolus
- − Infectious
  - • Septic encephalopathy can be a result of any infections other than primary CNS infections
  - • Symptoms may be owing to widespread multiorgan injury associated with the systemic inflammatory response
  - • Causes of septic encephalopathy
    - □ Bacteremia/sepis
    - □ Urinary tract infection/urosepsis
    - □ Pneumonia
    - □ Peritonitis
    - □ Bacterial endocarditis
- − Gastrointestinal
  - • Hepatic encephalopathy
    - □ Caused by cirrhosis of any cause, can be triggered or exacerbated by GI bleeding
    - □ EEG abnormalities can include bilaterally synchronous δ-waves, that are frequently biphasic
    - □ Asterixis: lapses of sustained muscle contraction. Can occur with other metabolic encephalopathies as well (including hypercapnia)
    - □ Magnetic resonance imaging (MRI) can show diffuse cerebral edema
    - □ Ammonia levels are often elevated
    - □ Liver function tests can be high, low or normal
    - □ Coagulopathy can result
    - □ Treatment
      - ◊ Prevent elevated ammonia concentrations
      - ◊ Dietary restrictions of protein
      - ◊ Antibiotics (such as neomycin) to suppress or eliminate urease-producing bowel bacteria
      - ◊ Lactulose from 30 to 50 mL PO/rectally qd to qid
      - ◊ Liver transplant has been successful in reversing encephalopathy and even coma
  - • Pancreatic insufficiency
- − Renal failure leading to uremia

- Endocrine causes
  - Thyroid disease
    □ Hypothyroidism
      ◊ "Myxedema coma": obtundation, nonpitting edema, hypothermia, hypoventilation, hypotension, and hypoglycemia
      ◊ Treated with thyroid replacement with cardiovascular and pulmonary supportadrenal insufficiency may coexist
    □ Hyperthyroidism
      ◊ Encephalopathy, hyperdynamic cardiac function (tachycardia, increased cardiac output and ejection fraction), decreased vascular resistance, arrythmias (afib, SVT), pulmonary compromise, and fever
      ◊ If suspected, therapy should be started immediately. Close monitoring, cardiovascular/pulmonary/fluid support, and rapid administration of antithyroid drugs and β-blockers
  - Acute adrenal failure
    □ Addisonian crisis from pituitary tumors, primary adrenal disease, adrenal suppression from chronic steroid therapy or rapid cessation of steroids
    □ Symptoms: obtundation with hyponatremia and hyperkalemia
    □ May follow infection, injury or surgery
    □ Diagnosis can be confirmed by random cortisol levels below 20 µg/dL; if in doubt, a cosyntropin stimulation test may be required
    □ Treatment: 100mg IV hydrocortisone followed by a 75–100 mg dose every 6 h, followed by an oral taper
      ◊ If planning a cosyntropin test but immediate treatment is needed, give dexamethasone 4 mg iv every 4 h instead of hydrocortisone, as dexamethasone will not interfere with the measurement of endogenous cortisol levels; when the test is complete, the patient can be tapered to hydrocortisone
  - Hypopituitarism
    □ Addison's disease
    □ Cushing's disease
  - Parathyroid disorders
    □ Hypoparathyroid
    □ Hyperparathyroid

- Porphyria
- Nutritional
  - Vitamin deficiency
    - □ Thiamine
      - ◊ Wernicke's encephalopathy
      - ◊ Ophthalmoplegia, ataxia, global confusion
      - ◊ Treatment: immediate administration of thiamine 50–100 mg IV or IV. This dose should be repeated daily until the patient resumes a normal diet and should be given before glucose-containing solutions
      - ◊ Korsakoff's psychosis
    - □ B_{12} deficiency
    - □ Folate deficiency
    - □ Pyridoxine deficiency
    - □ Nicotinic acid deficiency
  - Hypervitaminosis: A and D
- Body temperature: hypothermia, hyperthermia
- Acid-base disorders
- Cardiac: Arrythmia
- Errors of metabolism
  - Wilson's disease

Key Points

♦ Encephalopathy usually presents with nonfocal neurological exam as a result of diffuse cerebral disturbance
♦ Common and reversible etiologies should be investigated first (electrolytes, glucose, hypoxia, infection)
♦ Toxic and withdrawal syndromes occur commonly

Suggested Reading

American Psychiatric Association. *Diagnostic and Statistical Manual of Mental Disorders,* 4th edition. Washington, DC: American Psychiatric Association; 1994:123–133.

Aminoff MJ, ed. *Neurology and General Medicine,* 3rd edition. Philadelphia: Churchill Livingston;2001:593–615, 617–629, 631–644, 861–867, 1053–1067.

Bergeron N, Dubois MJ, Dumont M, et al. Intensive care delirium screening checklist: evaluation of a new screening tool. *Intensive Care Med* 2001;27:859–864.

Bergeron N, Skrobik Y, and Dubois MJ. (2002) Delirium in critically ill patients. *Crit Care* 2002;6(3):181–182.

Chen R and Young GB. Metabolic encephalopathies. *Baillieres Clin Neurol* 1996;5(3):577–598.

Ely EW, Gautam S, Margolin R, et al. The impact of delirium in the intensive care unit on hospital length of stay. *Intensive Care Medicine* 2001;27:1892–1900.

Ely EW, Margolin R, Francis J, et al. (2001) Evaluation of delirium in critically ill patients: validation of the confusion assessment method for the intensive care unit (CAM-ICU). *Crit Care Med* 2001;29(7): 1370–1379.

Marino PL, ed. *The ICU Book,* 2nd edition. Philadelphia: Lippincott, Williams and Wilkins;1998:779–793.

Naik-Tolani S, Oropello JM, and Benjamin E. (1999) Neurologic complications in the intensive care unit. *Clin Chest Med* 1999;20(2): 423–34, ix.

Rincon HG, Granados M, Unutzer J, et al. Prevalence, detection and treatment of anxiety, depression and delirium in the adult critical care unit. *Psychosomatics* 2001;42:391–396.

3 Intracerebral Hemorrhage

Romergryko G. Geocadin

Epidemiology

♦ The term intracerebral hemorrhage (ICH) is frequently used interchangeably with hemorrhagic strokes

♦ ICH encompasses the nontraumatic disorders that present with bleeding into the cranial vault

♦ Seen in 40,000–50,000 persons per year in the United States Worldwide incidence 10–20 cases/100,000

♦ More common in males, persons >55 yr of age and higher in certain ethic groups (blacks and Japanese)

♦ ICH accounts for approx10–15% of all strokes and has a higher morbidity and mortality than ischemic strokes. Only 38% of patients survive in the first year

Pathophysiology

♦ Nontraumatic ICH occurs at the following intracranial sites: Epidural, subdural, subarachnoid, intraparenchymal and intraventricular space

♦ From an etiologic standpoint ICH can be divided into "primary," most commonly associated with systemic hypertension and "secondary" caused by a clinically defined disorder other than hypertension (*see* Fig. 1 and Table 1)

♦ ICH results from rupture of the cerebral vasculature resulting from any or a combination of:

  – Increase in intraluminal pressure (hypertension)

  – Weakness of the blood vessel wall (vascular malformation and vasculopathies)

From: *Current Clinical Neurology: Handbook of Neurocritical Care*
Edited by: A. Bhardwaj, M. A. Mirski, J. A. Ulatowski © Humana Press Inc., Totowa, NJ

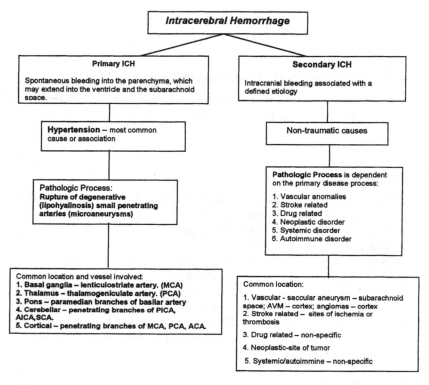

Fig. 1. Pathophysiologic features of intracerebral hemorrhage. (Adapted from Qureshi Al, Tuhrim S, Broderick JP, Batjer HH, Hondo H, and Hanley DF; 2001:1450–1460.)

    – Bleeding and coagulation problems (thrombocytopenia, anticoagulants and thrombolytics)

Clinical Presentation

♦ Symptoms and signs can be sudden and clinically devastating, such as those with massive intraparenchymal hemorrhage; or slow and initially nonspecific, such as those with subacute or chronic subdural hematoma

♦ High index of clinical suspicion in patients presenting with rapid onset of neurological deficit associated with abrupt deterioration in level of consciousness

Table 1
Common Etiology and Risk Factors for Intracranial Hemorrhage

1. Systemic hypertension
2. Vascular anomalies
   a. Intrancranial aneurysm
   b. Arteriovenous malformation
   c. Cavernous or venous angiomas
3. Cerebral vessel occlusion related
   a. Hemorrhagic conversion of ischemic stroke
   b. Cerebral venous thrombosis
4. Amyloid angiopathy
5. Drug related
   a. Anticoagulation (heparin and warfarin)
   b. Antiplatelets (aspirin, clopidogrel, ticlopidine, etc.)
   c. Thrombolytics (rTPA)
   d. Drug or substance abuse:
      i. Alcohol
      ii. Cocaine
6. Toxemia of pregnancy
7. Neoplastic disorders
   a. Primary intracranial tumor (i.e., Glioblastoma multiforme)
   b. Secondary tumor (metastasis)
      i. Renal cell carcinoma
      ii. Thyroid ca
      iii. Melanoma
      iv. Choriocarcinoma
      v. Lung carcinoma
8. Systemic disorders
   a. Hypertension (primary or secondary)
   b. Renal failure
   c. Liver failure
   d. Coagulopathy
   e. Hemolytic disorders
9. Autoimmune disorders
   a. Primary cerebral vasculitis
   b. Systemic collagen vascular disorders
10. Infections
    a. Mycotic aneurysm

♦ Reduction in the level of consciousness (LOC) may be a result of:
  – Intracranial pressure (ICP) elevation with global reduction in
  cerebral perfusion

- Mechanical compression of the brainstem and the impairment of the reticular activating system

♦ Supratentorial lesions affecting the cortical areas may be manifested as cortical dysfunction such as asphasia, neglect, hemiparesis, visual field defects or seizures

♦ Infratentorial lesions causing brain stem impairment and reduction in level of consciousness; cranial nerve dysfunction leading to diplopia, dysphagia and dysarthria and motor deficits

♦ A lesion in the cerebellum or its connections causes dysmetria, nystagmus and ataxia

♦ A hemorrhagic extension into the ventricles or a parenchymal hematoma compressing of the cerebrospinal fluid (CSF) pathways may lead to an obstructive hydrocephalus causing a reduction in the LOC secondary to elevated ICP

Diagnosis

♦ A nonenhanced head computerized tomography (CT) scan is still the preferred modality for rapid diagnosis. This test differentiates ICH from cerebral infarction

♦ Key findings on initial head CT scan that can affect the emergent management are initial hematoma size, supratentorial or infratentorial location, presence and extent of hydrocephalus, intraventricular extension, and midline shift or brain herniation

♦ Certain lesions are amenable to urgent surgical intervention such as acute hemorrhage into the epidural, subdural, subarachnoid spaces, and cerebellar lesions must also be taken into consideration

♦ Estimation of ICH volume on CT scan is valuable in management and prognosis in these patients. A rapid method to estimate parenchymal hematoma volume has been developed and validated

- "ABC" method estimates the volume as half the product of A, B, and C; where A is the greatest diameter of ICH on CT, B is the diameter perpendicular to A, and C is the thickness of the hematoma (based on the number of slices showing the hematoma multiplied by the slice thickness)

- It has been shown that a parenchymal hematoma size of more than 30 cc on initial head CT is associated with early neurological deterioration

♦ Additional diagnostic neuroimaging is necessary in patients with suspected vascular malformations. Timing of additional neuroimaging is balanced with the patient's clinical condition and the benefit from possible intervention, such as surgery

♦ Cerebral angiography is important in determining:
  – Arterial vascular malformation, especially in younger patients
    (<45 yr of age) without a history of hypertension
  – Intracranial aneurysms in those with predominance of blood in
    the subarachnoid space
♦ Magnetic resonance imaging (MRI) with gadolinium enhancement
and magnetic resonance angiography (MRA) may be helpful in
identifying other causes of the bleed such as tumor or vascular
malformation
♦ Evidence of recurrent hemorrhages also warrants additional neuroimaging. Some patients with negative imaging studies may benefit
from repeat imaging after 2–4 wk if the clinical circumstances continue to support a high likelihood for the hemorrhage to be the result
of a secondary cause

Management

♦ Can be divided into the interventions directed at the primary
problem (ICH) and secondary interventions directed at the effects
and complications of the hemorrhage
♦ *Primary* management of ICH is focused on three key factors (that
influence the initiation and termination of bleeding):
  – Intra-arterial pressure
  – Integrity of the vascular wall
  – Role of hemostatic factors (platelets and coagulation pathways).
  – Much of the emergent and life threatening injuries caused by
    ICH are in its secondary effects and complications
♦ *Secondary* effects and complications of ICH focuses on:
  – Mass effect of the actual hematoma and edema
  – ICP elevation from the mass effect or the obstruction of CSF
    pathways with hydrocephalus
  – Seizures

Considerations During Emergent Management

♦ Neurological status of these patients needs to be carefully monitored, ideally in an intensive care environment
♦ Active bleeding with continued hematoma expansion is the most
common cause of neurological deterioration during the initial hours
after the diagnosis. Hematoma expansion occurs in about (26% of
patients after the first CT scan and in another 12% within 20 h)
♦ About 25% of all patients with ICH who are initially alert may
deteriorate clinically with a reduction in LOC within 24 h of symp-

tom onset that is associated with a large hematoma size and hemorrhagic extension into the ventricle

♦ Other factors associated with neurologic deterioration include:
  - Re-hemorrhage
  - Associated cerebral edema
  - Hydrocephalus and ICP elevation
  - Seizures (especially with lesions in the cortex)

♦ The initial and emergent phase management focuses on rapid assessment of the adequacy of patient's airway, promoting adequate breathing and stabilizing the hemodynamic status

♦ Airway:
  - Patients with large ICH have increased likelihood of ICP elevation, coma, and loss of airway protection and need for endotracheal intubation
  - Evaluation of the patient's LOC and integrity of airway reflexes is important
  - During endotracheal intubation, sedation or general anesthesia prevents excessive elevations in systemic blood pressure occur that may further expand the hematoma. A delay in securing the airway may worsen injury secondary to hypoxemia, aspiration, and hypercapnia

♦ Breathing:
  - In patients with large ICH, consciousness and breathing may be impaired leading to hypoxia (pO_2 <60 mmHg) and hypercarbia (pCO_2 >50 mmHg). Both are systemically detrimental, and can cause ICP elevation from cerebral vasodilatation thus worsening cerebral perfusion
  - After securing the airway by intubation, adequate oxygenation and ventilation are facilitated. Therapeutic hyperventilation can be instituted when ICP elevation or cerebral herniation is actively ongoing. Prophylactic and excessive hyperventilation is harmful and not recommended

♦ Circulation:
  - Adequate vascular access for diagnosis and therapy is established
  - Placement of an arterial catheter for continuous blood pressure (BP) reading is recommended but intermittent noninvasive monitoring may be adequate
  - There is evidence that a reduction in cerebral perfusion pressure (CPP) (i.e., <70 mmHg) may lead to worsening of neurologi-

cal injury (CPP = mean arterial pressure minus ICP). The management of blood pressure is provided in a separate section below

– Cushing's syndrome consisting of intracranial hypertension with hypertension, bradycardia and rapid breathing must be promptly differentiated from essential hypertension alone, a common cause of ICH

♦ Diagnostics:
– Establish patient's history of bleeding, drug intake, especially use of warfarin and anti-platelets agents
– Any systemic or metabolic abnormalities, especially those that may predispose to more bleeding are corrected
– After hemodynamic and respiratory stabilization, rapid diagnostic and neuroimaging are undertaken
– Most important diagnostic differentiation is cerebral aneurysm and vascular malformation by MRA or conventional angiogram in patients who present atypically

Management of Primary Injury

♦ Blood pressure management:
– Systemic hypertension is commonly observed after hemorrhagic strokes
– The occurrence of elevated blood pressure after the bleed has been associated with hematoma expansion and poor outcome
– The precise management of elevated BP following ICH is hampered by the absence of well-controlled clinical trials
– In treating systemic hypertension, factors that lead to BP elevation are considered, such as agitation, chronic hypertension, ICP elevation (in association with Cushing response), and older patients
– Pharmacological reduction of mean arterial pressure (MAP) by 10–20 mmHg in patients with small to moderate ICH (1 cc to 45 cc vol) has no detrimental effect on global and peri-hematomal cerebral blood flow
– In patients with large ICH volume (>45 cc), the American Heart Association (AHA) provides the following guidelines for management of BP:
  • For patients with chronic hypertension maintain a mean arterial BP <130 mmHg

Table 2
Blood Pressure Management in Intracranial Hemorrhage

Agents for control of high blood pressure
   Labetalol: 5–100 mg/h by intermittent bolus of 10–40 mg iv or
      continuous drip at 2–8 mg/min
   Esmolol: 500 µg/kg load then 50–200 mcg/kg/min
   Enalaprilat: 0.625–1.2 mg iv q 6 h
   Hydralazine: 2.5–10 mg q 20 min
   Nitroprusside: 0.5–10 µg/kg/min
Agents for management of low blood pressure
   Volume replacement with isotonic saline or colloids (as appropriate)
   Vasopressors are recommended if hypotension persists after adequate
      im volume replacement. These agents can be titrated to the desired
      MAP (>90 mmHg)
   Phenylephrine: 2–10 µg/kg/min
   Dopamine: 2–20 µg/kg/min
   Norpinephrine: 0.05–0.2 µg/kg/min

- For patients with ICP elevation and ICP monitor, MAP is controlled to maintain a CPP >70 mmHg
- For those in post-operative period, MAP must be maintained <110 mmHg.
- Antihypertensive agents recommended for use are provided in Table 2 (Adapted from AHA Guidelines for Management of Spontaenous ICH, 1999).
– In those patients with low MAP, volume resuscitation with isotonic fluids is undertaken to maintain euvolemia. Volume status may be monitored with adjunctive measures such central venous pressure. If hypotension persists after adequate fluid resuscitation, continuous vasopressors (Table 2) are used to maintain a MAP >90 mmHg or ideally maintain a CPP >70 mmHg (if ICP monitoring is available)
♦ Surgical Considerations:
– Neurosurgical evacuation of an ICH is ideally undertaken with the least amount of brain injury, to reduce mass effect and limit other secondary injuries. However, a meta-analysis of three randomized controlled trials on the evacuation of supratentorial hematoma by open craniotomy showed that patients who underwent surgical evacuation had higher death and dependency rates as compared to best medical management (83 vs 70%). With the

APPROACH TO A PATIENT WITH INTRACEREBRAL HEMORRHAGE (ICH)

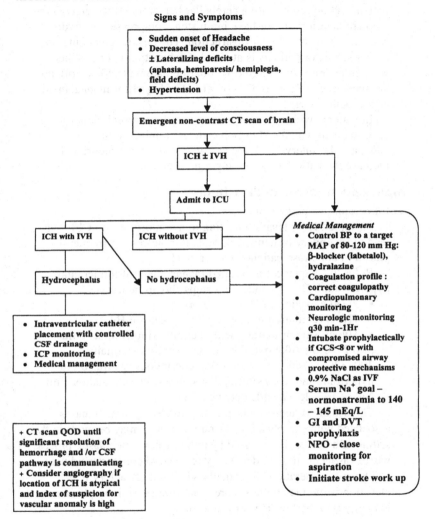

Fig. 2. Approach to a patient with intracerebral hemorrhage.

absence of a group benefit from surgical evacuation of hematoma, the surgical evacuation in the setting of a fast expanding hematoma to reverse herniation may be considered in individual patients in a few carefully selected cases

– Neurosurgical intervention however, is recommended in patients who present with a cerebellar hematoma (diameter >3 cm) who are deteriorating or have brain stem compression or hydrocephalus from ventricular obstruction. The best surgical outcome in this subset of patients is attained if evacuation is undertaken early in patients with large cerebellar hematoma (>40 cc vol) and Glasgow Coma Score (GCS) of <14 (*See* Fig. 3 for management of cerebellar ICH)

– In patients with secondary causes for the cerebral hemorrhage, such as aneurysm, AVM or hemorrhagic tumor, surgical or endovascular intervention are considered if the procedure will increase the patient's chance for a good outcome

Management of Secondary Injury

♦ Intracranial Hypertension

– Sustained ICP elevation leading to a compromise in CPP may lead to secondary ischemic injury. ICP monitors are frequently placed in comatose patients with an ICH

– Refer to Chapter 5 for detailed management of intracranial hypertensionl. Briefly, following steps should be taken:

• Head elevation to 30°above horizontal
• Hyperventilation to keep P_aCO_2 25–30 mmHg
• Hyperosmolar therapy with mannitol (intravenous bolus of 0.25–1.0 gm/kg q 4–6 h) to keep serum osmollaity 300–320 mOsm/L. Alternatively, continuous iv infusion of hypertonic saline (HS) (2 or 3% solution) to maintain serum Na^+ at 145–155 meq/L may be used

– The use of corticosteroids in ICH provides no benefit and is associated with complications. A rare exception may be made in the setting of a hemorrhage caused by an intracranial neoplastic process where vasogenic tumor edema may respond to corticosteroid use

– Other considerations in patients who have refractory ICP elevation is the metabolic suppression of brain activity pharmacologically with barbiturates or propofol

– Surgical management of persistent ICP elevation is considered emergently in patients with extension of ICH into the ventricle, compression of the CSF pathways leading to obstructive hydrocephalus, or impairment of the CSF outflow at the Pacchionian granulations causing communicating hydrocephalus. In these cases, CSF should be removed or diverted. An intraventricular catheter (IVC) with external drain is appropriate is the acute setting (*see* Chapter 11 for details)

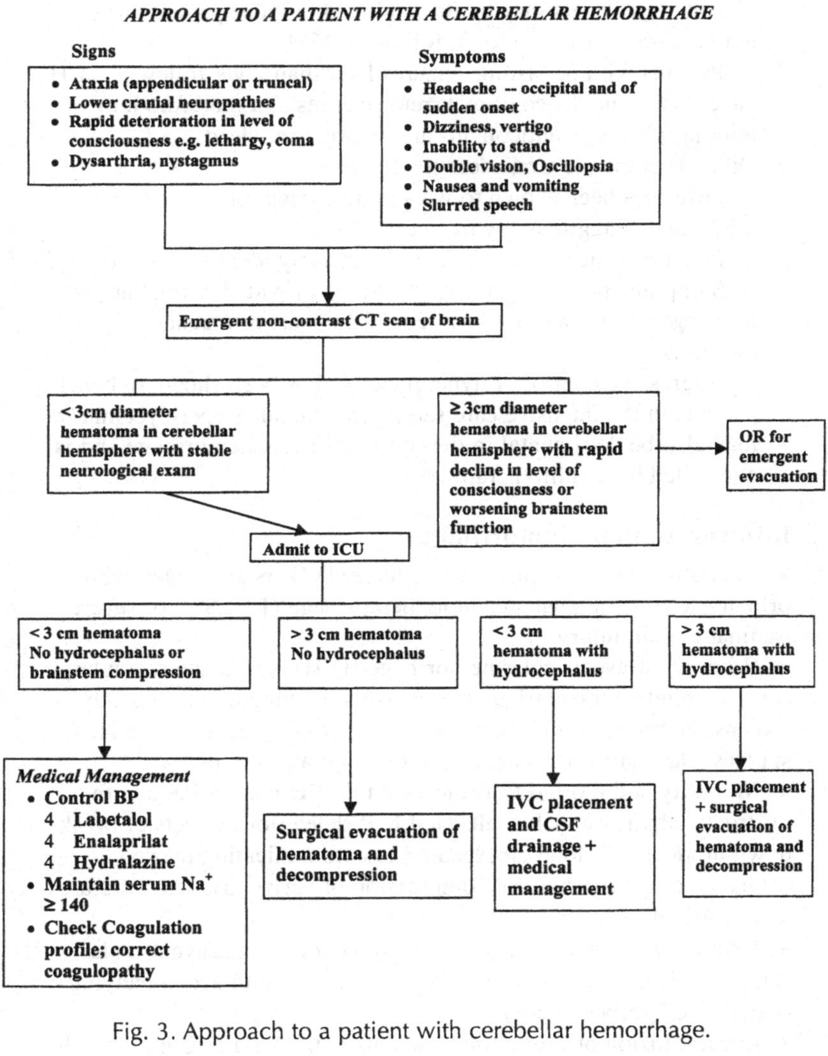

APPROACH TO A PATIENT WITH A CEREBELLAR HEMORRHAGE

Signs
- Ataxia (appendicular or truncal)
- Lower cranial neuropathies
- Rapid deterioration in level of consciousness e.g. lethargy, coma
- Dysarthria, nystagmus

Symptoms
- Headache -- occipital and of sudden onset
- Dizziness, vertigo
- Inability to stand
- Double vision, Oscillopsia
- Nausea and vomiting
- Slurred speech

Emergent non-contrast CT scan of brain

< 3cm diameter hematoma in cerebellar hemisphere with stable neurological exam

≥ 3cm diameter hematoma in cerebellar hemisphere with rapid decline in level of consciousness or worsening brainstem function

OR for emergent evacuation

Admit to ICU

<3 cm hematoma No hydrocephalus or brainstem compression

>3 cm hematoma No hydrocephalus

<3 cm hematoma with hydrocephalus

>3 cm hematoma with hydrocephalus

Medical Management
- Control BP
  4 Labetalol
  4 Enalaprilat
  4 Hydralazine
- Maintain serum Na$^+$ ≥ 140
- Check Coagulation profile; correct coagulopathy

Surgical evacuation of hematoma and decompression

IVC placement and CSF drainage + medical management

IVC placement + surgical evacuation of hematoma and decompression

Fig. 3. Approach to a patient with cerebellar hemorrhage.

♦ Seizures
  – A cortical hematoma increases the likelihood of seizures and most seizures occur within the first 24 h of the hemorrhage
  – The use of anticonvulsants to treat and as prophylaxis is justified in the acute phase of treatment

- Anticonvulsants may be discontinued in those patients who do not have seizure for a month following ICH
- Patients with persisting seizures later than 2 wk following ICH have higher incidence of recurrent seizures and therefore long term prophylactic anticonvulsant therapy is advised
♦ Other Therapeutic Considerations:
- Fever has been shown to worsen outcomes following brain injury and is aggressively treated
- Infectious causes for the fever are actively identified and treated
- Symptomatic management of fever is provided with pharmacologic agents (acetaminophen), cold infusions, or mechanical cooling (fans)
- Aggressive control of hyperglycemia has been shown to benefit patients in the intensive care setting in general. Hyperglycemia may also be detrimental in the setting of acute hemorrhage and is controlled by insulin therapy

Intraventricular Hemorrhage

♦ In adults, intraventricular hemorrhage (IVH) is associated with primary ICH (40%), subarcahnoid hemorrhage (10–28%) or severe traumatic brain injury
♦ Primary intraventricular hemorrhage (IVH) is rare and secondary causes include intraventricular neoplasms (meningionmas, ependymomas, metastatic tumors), cocaine use, pituitary apoplexy, eclampsia, vascular malformations, and rarely with aneurysms
♦ Mortality and morbidity is increased if IVH is associated with obstructive hydrocephalus, elevated ICP, deleterious effects of breakdown products of blood clot leading to communicating hydrocephalus, direct mechanical compression of periventricular structures, and ventriculitis
♦ Externalized CSF drainage via placement of an intraventricular cathether (IVC) is usually indicated (especially with accompanying obstructive hydrocephalus)
♦ Local infusion of thrombolytic agents (r-tPA) via IVC until resolution of clot and hydrocephalus is a promising new therapy. Results of prospective clinical trial are pending

Key Points

♦ Diagnosis and management in an intensice care unit (ICU) setting is paramount in patients with ICH

♦ Rapid neurologic deterioration may occur secondary to hematoma expansion, accompanying edema or hydrocephalus leading to elevated ICP

♦ Control of BP, anti-edema therapies, and ICP control are cornerstones of medical management

♦ Surgical evacuation can be life saving but is tailored for the individual patient depending on their age, size, and location of hematoma and co-morbidities

Suggested Reading

Qureshi AI, Tuhrim S, Broderick JP, Batjer HH, Hondo H, and Hanley DF. Spontaneous intracerebral hemorrhage. *N Engl J Med.* 2001;344:1450–1460.

Broderick JP, Adams HP, Jr., Barsan W, et al. Guidelines for the management of spontaneous intracerebral hemorrhage: A statement for healthcare professionals from a special writing group of the Stroke Council, American Heart Association. *Stroke* 1999;30:905–915.

Brott T, Thalinger K, and Hertzberg V. Hypertension as a risk factor for spontaneous intracerebral hemorrhage. *Stroke* 1986;17:1078–1083.

Brott T, Broderick J, Kothari R, et al. Early hemorrhage growth in patients with intracerebral hemorrhage. *Stroke* 1997;28:1–5.

Broderick JP, Brott TG, Duldner JE, Tomsick T, and Huster G. Volume of intracerebral hemorrhage. A powerful and easy-to-use predictor of 30-day mortality. *Stroke* 1993;24:987–993.

Mayer SA, Sacco RL, Shi T, and Mohr JP. Neurologic deterioration in noncomatose patients with supratentorial intracerebral hemorrhage. *Neurology* 1994;44:1379–1384.

Qureshi AI, Suri MA, Safdar K, Ottenlips JR, Janssen RS, amd Frankel MR. Intracerebral hemorrhage in blacks. Risk factors, subtypes, and outcome. *Stroke* 1997;28:961–964.

Powers WJ, Zazulia AR, Videen TO, et al. Autoregulation of cerebral blood flow surrounding acute (6 to 22 hours) intracerebral hemorrhage. *Neurology* 2001;57:18–24.

Hankey GJ and Hon C. Surgery for primary intracerebral hemorrhage: is it safe and effective? A systematic review of case series and randomized trials. *Stroke* 1997;28:2126–2132.

Naff NJ and Tuhrim S. Intraventricular hemorrhage in adults: Complications and treatment. *New Horiz* 1997;5:359–363.

4   Subarachnoid Hemorrhage

Anish Bhardwaj

Epidemiology of Subarachnoid Hemorrhage (SAH)

♦ Traumatic brain injury is the most common cause of blood in the subarchnoid space

♦ Rupture of intracranial (saccular or berry) aneurysm is the most common cause of nontraumatic spontaneous subarachnoid hemorrhage (SAH)

♦ Prevalence of intracranial aneurysms in the general population in the United States is approx 0.5–1.0%

♦ Prevalence of intracranial aneurysms in angiographic studies approx 3.5–6.0%

♦ Risk of aneurysmal rupture is approx 1.9%/yr

♦ Incidence of SAH is approx 6–25/100,000/yr in the United States.

♦ More common in females (F:M, 3:2), peaks in the sixth decade of life; before the 40 yr of age it is predominantly a disorder in males.

♦ 24-h mortality approx 25%

♦ 30-d mortality approx 45%

♦ SAH represents approx 4.5% of stroke mortality

♦ Risk factors for rupture include size (>7 mm), symptomatic aneurysms and gender (females > males)

♦ Smoking is the only risk factor that has consistently been identified with aneurysmal SAH

♦ Other associated risk factors for aneurysmal SAH:
- – Hypertension
- – Heavy alcohol consumption
- – Cocaine and amphetamine use
- – Oral contraceptive use

From: *Current Clinical Neurology: Handbook of Neurocritical Care*
Edited by: A. Bhardwaj, M. A. Mirski, J. A. Ulatowski © Humana Press Inc., Totowa, NJ

- Pregnancy or menopause (less clear role)
- Familial and hereditary factors
  - Polycystic kidney disease (autosomal dominant form)
  - Marfan's syndrome
  - Ehlers–Danlos type IV
  - Neurofibromatosis (type I)
  - Pseudoxanthoma elasticum
  - α-1-antitrypsin deficiency
  - Sickle cell disease
- ◆ Nonaneurysmal causes of SAH:
  - Head trauma
  - Arteriovenous malformations
  - Substance abuse (cocaine, amphetamines)
  - Arterial dissection
  - Myomoya disease
  - Idiopathic perimesencephalic SAH
  - Coagulopathy

Clinical Presentation of SAH

◆ Sudden onset of severe cataclysmic headache (approx 70% of patients)

◆ Nausea, vomiting, neck discomfort, photophobia, and phonophobia (signs of meningeal irritation)

◆ Sudden loss of consciousness (up to approx 45% of patients), attributed to decrease in cerebral perfusion pressure (CPP) or malignant cardiac arrhythmias

◆ A warning leak ("sentinel" hemorrhage in approx 70% of patients); its presence warrants a high index of suspicion

◆ Signs of SAH:
  - Depends on severity (Hunt–Hess Grade)
    - Grade I: asymptomatic or mild headache
    - Grade II: moderate to severe headache, nuchal rigidity, with or without cranial nerve deficits
    - Grade III: confusion, lethargy or mild focal symptoms
    - Grade IV: stupor and/or hemiparesis
    - Grade V: comatose and/or extensor posturing
  - Changes in vital signs:
    - Hypertension
    - Cardiac arrhythmias
    - Changes in respiratory pattern

- Focal neurological signs:
  - Occulomotor palsy (internal carotid artery [ICA]/posterior communicating artery aneurysm)
  - Paraparesis (anterior cerebral artery aneurysm)
  - Hemiparesis, aphasia, and neglect (middle cerebral artery aneurysm)
  - Binasal hemianopsia may occur with enlarging supraclinoid ICA aneurysm
- Signs of meningeal irritation:
  - Nuchal rigidity
  - Photophobia, phonophobia
  - Kernig's and Brudzunski's sign
- Subhyaloid hemorrhages on fundoscopic examination
♦ Mimics of SAH:
  - Migraine or tension headache
  - Viral meningitis
  - Head trauma
  - Sinusitis
  - Cervical disk disease
  - Alcohol/drug intoxication
  - Hypertensive encephalopathy
  - Ischemic stroke, transient ischemic attack
♦ Misdiagnosis of SAH
  - Occurs in 20–25% of patients with SAH
  - Most likely to occur in alert patients with only headache (HA) and with normal levels of consciousness or focal neurological signs
  - Occurs frequently in patients with chronic HA syndromes

Diagnostic Tests

♦ Noncontrast computed tomography (CT) of the brain is the diagnostic study of choice (85–90 % sensitivity)
  - Location of the clot seen on CT can be predictive of the location of the ruptured aneurysm
    - Fisher grading system is based on the CT appearance of blood in the subarachnoid space
      - Grade I: no SAH on CT scan
      - Grade II: broad diffusion of subarachnoid blood, no clots, and no layers of blood >1 mm
      - Grade III: either localized clots in the subarachnoid space or layers of blood >1 mm

       □ Grade IV: intraventricular and intracerebral blood present,
       in absence of significant subarachnoid blood
♦ If the CT is negative for SAH, a lumbar puncture is mandatory for
presence of blood or xanthochromia in the cerebrospinal fluid (CSF)
♦ Four vessel cerebral angiography remains the gold standard
    – Early angiography is recommended
    – Nonionic contrast material has less osmotic load and fewer
adverse reactions. Patients with contrast allergies can be pretreated
with steroids and benadryl
    – Digital subtraction techniques are preferred
    – Angiographic details to be delineated for appropriate treatment
strategies include:
      • Aneurysmal size
      • Orientation
      • Presence of neck
      • Irregularity in the fundus
      • Presence/absence of vasospasm
    – A conventional angiogram may not reveal an aneurysm
(10–30% of cases) because of:
      • Thrombus within the aneurysmal pouch
      • Vasospasm
      • Poor technique
      • Compression by an extravascular clot
    – May require repeat angiography, usually in 2 wk, that reveals
an aneurysm in 10–20% of cases.
    – In cases of a pretruncal (perimesencephalic) nonaneurysmal
SAH, where blood is limited in front of the brainstem, sparing the
ventricles and the lateral sylvian fissures, a second angiogram is
not indicated
♦ Other alternative diagnostic methods:
    – Helical computed tomographic angiography (CTA) provides
multiplanar views or three-dimensional (3-D) maximum intensity
projection images (sensitivity of 77–97% and specificity of
87–100%). May be used in an unstable patient that requires surgery before an angiogram can be performed
    – Magnetic resonance angiography (MRA), either as a 3-D time of
flight or 3-D phase contrast technique. Sensitivity depends on the
aneurysm size (higher for aneurysm >5 mm)
    – If SAH is more diffuse and repeat angiogram is negative, other
causes of SAH should be considered including:

- Trauma: usually has more peripheral distribution in subarachnoid space
- Cervical medullary arterial venous fistulas
- Spinal arteriovenous malformations
- Coagulation disorders
- Cocaine and amphetamine use
- Sickle cell disease
- Magnetic resonance imaging (MRI) of the brain and spinal cord is warranted to exclude any other vascular abnormalities

◆ Postoperative angiogram is usually done following aneurysmal clipping to demonstrate correct clip placement, distal and small perforator vessel patency, and the presence of vasospasm

Preoperative Medical Management of SAH

◆ Admit patient to a monitored critical care setting
◆ Assess level of consciousness
- Prophylactic endotracheal intubation for airway protection (GCS ≤8; Hunt–Hess Scale >3)
- Use general anesthetic induction to blunt the hemodynamic stress of laryngoscopy
◆ Blood Pressure Control
- Maintain 5–10% of premorbid values (if known) or systolic blood pressure (SBP) <150, diastolic blood pressure (DBP) <80, MAP <110 mmHg with the following antihypertensive agents
  - Labetalol, 10–40 mg iv Q 15–30 min
  - Enalaprilat 0.625–1.25 mg IV Q 6 h
  - Hydralazine 10–20 mg IV Q 20 min
◆ Seizure Prevention
- Phenytoin 18–20 mg/Kg IV load, then 300 mg/d
◆ Vasospasm Prophylaxis
- Nimodipine 60 mg Q 4 h PO/NGT
◆ Hydration
- Normal saline at 1–2 mL/Kg/h
◆ Analgesia and Sedation
- Morphine sulfate, 1–4 mg IV Q 1 h
- Fentanyl 25–50 µg IV Q 30min
◆ Steroids
- Dexamethasone 4–8 mg Q 6 h IV or orally
- Used preoperatively only and their use is controversial

♦ Gastrointestinal (GI) prophylaxis
  – H$_2$ antagonists (ranitidine 150 mg PO bid or 50 mg IV bid) or
  sucralfate (1 g PO Q 6 h) or Omeprazole (5 mg PO bid)

Timing of Aneurysmal Clipping

♦ Early surgery is favored and recommended for the following reasons:
  – To prevent rebleeding (occurs in approx 4% of patients within
  the first 24 h)
  – Better prevention of vasospasm (by intra-operative removal of
  the clot or injection of thrombolytics, like rtPA or more aggressive
  treatment with hypervolemic, hypertensive, and hemodilution
  (triple H) therapy
  – To prevent or treat hydrocephalus by mechanically removing the
  subarachnoid blood or any associated intraparenchymal hematoma
♦ Delayed surgery is considered in:
  – Complicated aneurysms (basilar bifurcation aneurysm or giant
  aneurysm with a diameter ≥2.5 cm)
  – Older patients or those in poor medical condition
♦ Early endovascular treatment with Guglielmi detachable coils (GDC)
is an alternative in high-risk patients (*see* "endovascular procedures")

Neuroradiological Endovascular Procedures

♦ Coil embolization has been proven feasible in the treatment of
ruptured aneurysms. Comparison studies with aneurysmal clipping
are forthcoming
♦ Complications such as perforation, distal migration, or parent
vessel thrombosis occur in up to approx 30% of patients undergoing
GDC placement
♦ Best results are obtained in small aneurysms, with narrow neck
(<4 mm), and in those with steep angle to the blood flow
♦ Multiple coils increase the risk for complications but improve
obliteration of aneurysm
♦ In addition to coiling, when the aneurysm is partially obliterated,
surgery may be performed at a later time, with reduced brain swelling

Perioperative Anesthesia Considerations

♦ Detailed preoperative evaluation of patient
  – Discussion with the neurosurgeon is required in order to
  achieve the primary goals:
    • Preventing aneurysmal re-rupture by minimizing hyperten-
    sive episodes, anxiety, and pain
    • Decrease brain swelling

- Manage elevated intracranial pressure (ICP)
- Avoid cerebral ischemia
- Avoid systemic complications
♦ General anesthetic considerations:
  - Ventilation, oxygenation, and tight hemodynamic control
  - Avoidance of systolic hypertension and coughing (or bucking on the endotracheal tube) that may cause re-rupture of the aneurysm
  - Preoperative considerations
    - Careful preoperative review of systems and co-existing diseases such as hypertension and pulmonary and cardiac disease
    - Preoperative neurologic status may influence the choice of anesthetic as brain injury lessens the need for deep anesthesia, except at the time of intubation
♦ Emergence from anesthesia
  - Although control of ventilation and hemodynamics are of paramount concern during emergence, the ability to perform a neurologic exam as soon as possible cannot be over emphasized
  - Hypertension and tachycardia can be managed with short acting agents such as esmolol, nitroprusside, and labetalol
  - Coughing or bucking on the endotracheal tube can be managed with intravenous lidocaine (1.5 mg/kg) or an additional 25–50 μg of iv fentanyl. After full reversal of the neuromuscular blockade, the patient can be extubated shortly after demonstrating the ability to follow simple commands such as moving all four extremities
  - Patients who were stuporous prior to induction should be left intubated and have their neuromuscular blockade reversed to allow a neurologic exam. Supplemental narcotics and assisting or controlling ventilation allow a greater tolerance of the endotracheal tube while still permitting a useful neurologic exam
  - Alternate approach is to reverse neuromuscular blockade and allow slow emergence from GA while the patient remains intubated
  - The patient can then be evaluated and extubated in the next 1–2 h in the ICU under controlled conditions following emergence from anesthesia
  - If sedation for maintaining endotraceal tube is necessary, narcotics for pain control with fentanyl and low-dose sedation with propofol suffices

Aneurysmal Rebleeding

♦ Aneurysmal re-rupture is a significant cause of morbidity and mortality (up to 75%) following SAH

♦ For unclipped aneurysms the risk of rebleeding is 4% during the first day after SAH, decreasing to 1.5%/d after 2 d and reaching a plateau of 2–4%/yr after 6 mo
♦ Postulated to be secondary to breakdown in peri-aneurysmal clot Uncontrolled hypertension may play a role
♦ Clipped aneurysms can also rebleed, but the risk is considerably less
♦ Rebleeding may manifest as an acute change in neurological status (increased headaches, nausea and vomiting, depressed level of consciousness), Cushing's response (increased ICP followed by compensatory increase in blood pressure), and drainage of fresh blood from an indwelling intraventricular catheter
♦ Diagnosis is confirmed with an emergent CT scan and comparison with previous studies

Seizures

♦ Occur in 10–25% of patients with SAH
♦ Immediate seizures or posturing may be seen in up to 25% of patients at the onset of SAH
♦ May be confused with "posturing" seen in high grade patients with SAH
♦ Prophylactic anticonvulsants, though controversial, are recommended. Phenytoin is the agent of choice
♦ Seizures may complicate patient's status by propagating secondary brain injury through rebleeding, hypertension or hypoxia/acidosis
♦ Increased incidence of seizures may occur peri-operatively in patients with aneurysms in middle cerebral artery (MCA) distribution, with intra-operative retraction of the temporal lobe, rebleeding, intracerebral hemorrhage, vasospasm leading to delayed ischemia, especially in the MCA aneurysm location

Hydrocephalus

♦ Acute
  – Occurs within 24 h of aneurysmal bleeding
  – Usually obstructive (noncommunicating) due to impedance of CSF flow, usually at the foramina or aqueduct from large clots within the ventricular system or from external compression of CSF pathways
  – Abrupt onset of lethargy, coma, or stupor
  – Emergent CT scan without contrast should be performed to differentiate rebleeding from hydrocephalus. Absence of lateralizing features on neurological exam is suggestive of hydrocephalus

APPROACH TO A PATIENT WITH PRIMARY SAH

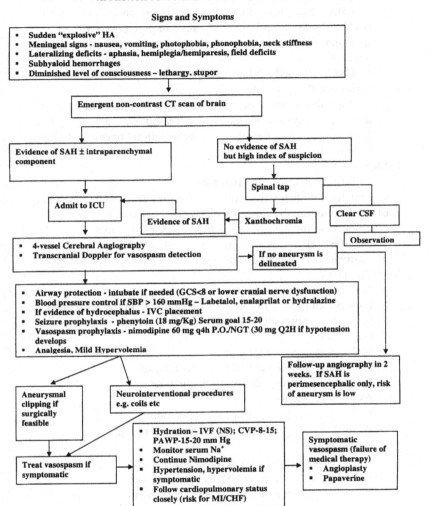

Fig. 1. Approach to a patient with primary SAH. Adapted from Varelas, Bhardwaj, and Eleff, 2000.

- Requires intraventricular catheter placement for CSF drainage
  - Extreme caution during insertion of intraventricular catheter (IVC). Should not relieve CSF pressure precipitously (and transmural pressure) that may cause re-rupture of an unclipped aneurysm
  - CSF is drained against an adjustable height fluid column resistance ("pop-off")
  - After the patient's mental status improves, the resistance of the draining system is gradually increased, with a goal of readjusting or priming the arachnoid granulation "opening" to higher pressures
- ◆ Subacute
  - 24 h to 7 d post-aneurysmal rupture
  - Usually nonobstructive (communicating) as a result of blockage of arachnoid granulations with blood products or CSF flow obstruction in the basal cisterns from large blood clots
  - Manifests clinically with impaired vertical gaze, memory impairment, gait abnormalities, intellectual decline, and progressive lethargy
  - May require lumbar drain/serial spinal taps
  - Extreme caution with lumbar CSF drainage in the presence of an unclipped aneurysm (concern for re-rupture)
- ◆ Delayed (late)
  - >10 d post-aneurysmal rupture
  - Frequently nonobstructive (communicating)
  - May require lumbar drain/serial spinal taps
  - Associated factors:
    - The presence of hydrocephalus on admission CT
    - High Fisher grade and intraventricular blood
    - Older age
    - Decreased level of consciousness on admission
    - Prehemorrhagic (premorbid) hypertension
  - Up to 20% of patients may require permanent CSF diversion with ventriculoperitoneal or ventriculopleural shunt within the first 30 d of SAH

Cerebral Vasospasm

- ◆ Angiographically demonstrated vasospasm may occur in 60–75% of patients with SAH
- ◆ Clinical neurological signs from delayed cerebral ischemia occurs in only one third of patients with SAH

♦ Usual presentation: new, gradual, or stepwise neurologic deficits, corresponding to cerebral vascular territory

♦ Characteristically occurs 4 through 21 d (peak incidence d 7 through 11)

♦ Best predictor for the development of vasospasm is the amount of blood detected on head CT (Fisher Grade) within the first 3 d after SAH (i.e., thicker the clot on CT the grater the incidence and severity of vasospasm)

♦ Is a proliferative vasculopathy

♦ Variety of vasoactive mediators have been implicated in the pathogenesis of cerebral vasospasm:
  – Oxyhaemoglobin
  – Free radicals
  – Prostaglandins through activation of protein kinase C
  – Decreased action of nitric oxide
  – Vasoconstrictive peptides like endothelin
  – Inflammatory immune mediators (e.g., ICAM-1)

♦ Serial neurologic examinations with ancillary tests are used for monitoring vasospasm

♦ Transcranial Doppler (TCD) provides:
  – Easy, noninvasive, bedside evaluation of blood flow velocities (BFV)
  – Not an absolute measure of cerebral blood flow
  – BFV >200 cm/s indicates severe vasospasm and correlates with severe angiographic vasospasm and usually precedes the development of ischemic symptoms.
  – Increase of BFV of 50 cm/s over a period of 24 h is a predictor of severe vasospasm
  – Careful interpretation of TCD results is needed when insonating the ACAs because they correlate less with angiographic vasospasm
  – Insonating intracranial vessels may not be possible due to lack of "windows" because of skull thickness in some patients
  – Inter-operator variability of approx 10% exists: Ideally a single operator should follow through repeated tests on the same patient

♦ Other methods that assess the cerebral blood flow (CBF), either qualitative (SPECT) or quantitative (PET), have not found wide applicability because of their high cost and time constraints

♦ Angiography remains the gold standard and can detect diffuse or focal vasospasm. MRA has suboptimal sensitivity for detecting vasospasm

♦ Medical treatment of vasospasm consists of the prophylactic administration of the dihydropyridine class of calcium channel antagonists (nimodipine, nicardipine) because they:
- Readily cross the blood–brain barrier
  • Improve outcome without resolving angiographic vasospasm. Postulated to provide benefit through collateral dilatation or their neuroprotective effects (impeding the excitotoxic cascade)
  • Nimodipine administration should be started immediately after SAH and continued for 21 d.
  • Use of nicardipine is not recommended because of its blood-pressure lowering effects

♦ Hypervolemic hypertensive hemodilutional (triple H) therapy improves neurologic status in 60% of the patients and decreases incidence of major neurologic deficit or death to <7%. Should be started only after the aneurysm is secured

♦ Hemodilution aims at decreasing blood viscosity and increasing CBF, without compromising tissue oxygen delivery. Optimal hematocrit is 30–33% and can usually be reached by simply not transfusing the patient during or following the operation or by instituting hypervolemic therapy

♦ Hypervolemic therapy should be instituted by administering isotonic fluids (0.9% saline), colloid or transfusion of blood products if appropriate

♦ Pulmonary edema is a complication. The patient should therefore be monitored with a Swan–Ganz catheter, aiming at a pulmonary artery wedge pressure (PAWP) of 14–18 mmHg. Because central venous pressure often correlates poorly with PAWP, its use in guiding therapy may be limited

♦ If delayed ischemic deficits do not improve, induced hypertension should be used to increase CBF, which is pressure dependent in many patients as a result of impaired autoregulation

♦ Vasopressors (phenylephrine) or inopressors (dopamine, epinephrine, dobutamine) are used to maintain the MAP and cardiac output high enough to reverse the deficit without untoward side effects

♦ Vasopressors should be tapered as soon as the neurologic deficits are reversed and hypervolemia can sustain the improvement solely

♦ If neurologic deficits cannot be reversed, HHH therapy can be continued for days, with careful monitoring of cardiac, pulmonary, and renal function as well as peripheral tissue and gut ischemia (lactate levels)

♦ Balloon angioplasty is recommended in cases of refractory vasospasm to HHH therapy
  – It mechanically dilates the proximal portions of the vessels, thus increasing distal CBF
  – Its effect is long lasting and can be safely used in patients with clipped aneurysms
  – Early procedure following recognition of failed medical therapy is recommended
  – Complications include arterial rupture and displacement of the clips
♦ Papaverine with or without angioplasty is utilized occasionally as a supraselective intra-arterial infusion.
  – It dilates the vessels by inhibiting cAMP and cGMP in smooth muscle cells
  – It can be used when vasospasm is diffuse or the vessel anatomy is suboptimal for angioplasty (the vessel is sharply angulated)
  – Effects are short lived and repeat infusions may be required
  – May also lead to increased ICP, tachycardia, arrhythmias, and occasionally seizures

Volume and Osmolar Disturbances

♦ Volume contraction and negative sodium balance develops in 30–50% of patients with SAH
♦ Hyponatremia that occurs in up to approx 30% of patients with SAH can be caused by:
  – Cerebral salt wasting syndrome
    • Probably because of elevated atrial natriuretic factor, decreased rennin, and aldosterone
    • Presents with natriuresis, hypovolemia, and hyponatremia
    • Should be treated aggressively with hypertonic saline solutions (1.5–3% hypertonic saline), if $Na^+ \leq 125$ or $Na^+ \leq 130$ especially in the presence of vasospasm or cerebral edema
  – Syndrome of inappropriate secretion of antidiuretic hormone (SIADH)
    • Less likely than cerebral salt wasting in the setting of SAH
    • Leads to free water retention, normo- or hypervolemia, and dilutional hyponatremia
    • Treated with fluid restriction, an approach that is contraindicated in patients with vasospasm

Cardiac Complications

♦ Affects up to 50% of patients following SAH
♦ Cardiac arrhythmias occur in up to approx 90% of patients with SAH and attributed to high levels of circulating catecholamines
♦ Most common manifestations include global electrocardiographic abnormalities (T wave inversion, ST segment depression, U waves, and QT interval prolongation), arrhythmias (bradyarrhythmias, premature complexes, supra or ventricular tachycardias). Elevated cardiac enzymes and echocardiographic ventricular wall abnormalities (10% of patients) suggest subendocardial ischemia
♦ Potentially life-threatening arrhythmias (asystole, ventricular tachycardia, and hemodynamically significant atrial fibrillation) occur in <5% of patients.
♦ "Neurogenic cardiac stun" may occur at presentation in high-grade patients with SAH
♦ Usually occur in the first 48 h following SAH and resolve over 1–2 wk
♦ Etiology of these cardiac manifestations are probably a consequence of increased sympathetic tone and catecholamine secretion. Early institution of β-blockers may reverse these changes
♦ Electrolyte abnormalities (hypokalemia, hyponatremia, hypophosphatemia, and hypomagnesemia) should be corrected during triple-H therapy

Pulmonary Complications

♦ Account for up to approx 50% of medical mortality after SAH
♦ Pneumonia frequently (from aspiration), is a result of decreased level of consciousness and poor airway reflexes, especially in patients with higher Hunt and Hess score
♦ Patients are also more prone to the development of neurogenic pulmonary edema that affects 2% of patients who are comatose
  – Neurogenic pulmonary edema presents with dyspnea, frothy, pink airway secretions, containing high protein. Increased positive-end expiratory pressure (PEEP) and FiO_2 are needed to correct the hypoxemia.
  – It is postulated to be caused by increased permeability of the pulmonary vascular epithelium secondary to massive sympathetic outflow
  – Contrasts with pulmonary edema with low protein content, usually a result of left ventricular failure and increased pulmonary

capillary wedge pressure. Often precipitated by iatrogenic hypervolemic therapy

Infectious Complications

♦ CNS infections:
  – Iatrogenic from an IVC placement
  – Occasionally from craniotomy during aneurysmal clipping
  – Use of prophylactic antibiotics is controversial with an IVC *in situ*, though they are widely used with agents that are effective against skin flora (e.g., Oxacillin 1 g IV q6h, clindamycin 500 mg IV q 8h, Ancef 1 g IV q6h)
  – Specific treatment of CNS infections depends on gram stain, culture, and sensitivity of CSF
  – With a high index of suspicion for infection, surveillance CSF cell count and cultures are recommended with an IVC or lumbar drain *in situ.*
  – If index of suspicion is low for infection, IVC may be left *in situ* for up to 2 wk.
♦ Systemic Infections:
  – Occur more commonly in patients with SAH
  – Pulmonary infections
    • Aspiration pneumonia that may be confirmed by a chest radiograph, Gram-negative stain, and sputum culture
  – Urinary tract infections with Gram-negative organisms in patients with in-dwelling catheters are commonly implicated. Treatment with appropriate antibiotics following Gram stain and culture are recommended
  – Incidence of sinusitis can be reduced by placing tracheal and gastric tubes via the oral route

Nutritional Support and Gastrointestinal Complications

♦ Patients with SAH are in a markedly catabolic state
♦ Enteral route is preferred and recommended to maintain the structural integrity of the intestinal villi
♦ GI bleeding occurs in approx 6% of patients with SAH secondary to stress ulcers or gastritis. Steroid use may exacerbate GI hemorrhage
♦ Cytoprotective agents should be given for GI prophylaxis:
  – H_2 antagonists (ranitidine 150 mg PO bid or 50 mg IV bid)
  – Sucralfate (1 g PO Q 6 h)
  – Omeprezole (5 mg PO bid).

♦ Ileus can be prevented with agents that enhance GI motility (reglan 10 mg IV/PO Q 6 h)

Deep Venous Thrombosis and Pulmonary Embolism

♦ Patients with SAH are at a high risk for deep venous thrombosis and subsequent pulmonary embolism (PE) resulting from prolonged immobility

♦ Sequential compression devices in the lower extremities should be used preoperatively

♦ Prior to aneurysmal clipping and in the immediate postoperative period, PE is usually managed with placement of a filter in the inferior vena cava

♦ One week following aneurysmal clipping and craniotomy, anticoagulation with heparin should be used (5000 U sq bid or tid)

Key Points

♦ High index of clinical suspicion is paramount in making a prompt diagnosis of SAH

♦ Early diagnostic tests and early aneurysmal clipping or coiling is the standard of care

♦ Nimodipine and hypertensive and hypervolemic therapy remain the principle medical therapies for cerebral vasospasm to prevent delayed ischemic deficits

♦ Balloon angioplasty can be performed early following failure of medical therapy for cerebral vasospasm

♦ Aggressive prevention and treatment of medical complications is paramount for good recovery

Suggested Reading

Bejjani GK, Bank WO, Olan WJ, and Sekhar LN. The efficacy and safety of angioplasty for cerebral vasospasm after subarachnoid hemorrhage. *Neurosurgery* 1998;42(5):979–986; discussion 986–987.

Fisher CM, Kistler JP, and Davis JM. Relation of cerebral vasospasm to subarachnoid hemorrhage visualized by computerized tomographic scanning. *Neurosurgery* 1980;6(1):1–9.

Graves VB, Strother CM, Duff TA, and Perl J. 2nd. Early treatment of ruptured aneurysms with Guglielmi detachable coils: effect on subsequent bleeding. *Neurosurgery* 1995;37(4):640–647; discussion 647–648.

Lanzino G. and Kassell NF. Surgical treatment of the ruptured aneurysm. Timing. *Neurosurg Clin N Am* 1998;9(3):541–548.

Mayberg MR, Batjer HH, Dacey R, et al. Guidelines for the management of aneurysmal subarachnoid hemorrhage. A statement for healthcare professionals from a special writing group of the Stroke Council, American Heart Association. *Stroke* 1994;25(11):2315–2328.

McKhann GM, 2nd and Le Roux PD. Perioperative and intensive care unit care of patients with aneurysmal subarachnoid hemorrhage. *Neurosurg Clin N Am* 1998;9(3):595–613.

Newell DW and Winn HR. Transcranial Doppler in cerebral vasospasm. *Neurosurg Clin N Am* 1990;1(2):319–328.

Solenski NJ, Haley EC, Jr, Kassell NF, et al. Medical complications of aneurysmal subarachnoid hemorrhage: a report of the multicenter, cooperative aneurysm study. Participants of the Multicenter Cooperative Aneurysm Study [*see* comments]. *Crit Care Med* 1995;23(6): 1007–1017.

Suarez JI, Qureshi AI, Parekh PD, et al. Administration of hypertonic (3%) sodium chloride/acetate in hyponatremic patients with symptomatic vasospasm following subarachnoid hemorrhage *J Neurosurg Anesthesiol* 1999;11(3):178–184.

Varelas P, Bhardwaj A, and Eleff SM. Critical care management of subarachnoid hemorrhage. Brunei *Int Med J* 2000;2:77–91.

Bleck TP. Medical management of subarachnoid hemorrhage. *New Horiz* 1997;5:387–396.

Hunt WE and Hess RM. Surgical risk as related to time of intervention in the repair of intracranial aneurysma. *J Neurosurg* 1968;28(1):14–20.

5 Cerebral Edema and Intracranial Hypertension

Anish Bhardwaj

Intracranial Vault: Physiological Concepts

♦ Contents of intracranial vault:
- Brain (80%)
- Cerebrospinal fluid (CSF) (10%; approx 75–100 mL)
- Blood (10%) (75 mL)

♦ Normal intracranial pressure (ICP) 5–15 mm Hg. Transient increments with valsalva, coughing, sneezing

♦ An increase in any of the three components is at the expense of the other two components to maintain a normal ICP initially. Compensatory mechanisms include (in order):
- Displacement of CSF from the cranial vault
- Displacement of blood
- Displacement of brain substance ("herniation")

♦ ICP rises exponentially with small increments in intracranial volume beyond a certain threshold (poor intracranial elastance [Δpressure/Δvolume])

ICP Monitoring Techniques

♦ Fluid coupled devices with external transducer:
- Intraventricular catheter (IVC):
  • Most reliable and widely used technique
  • Can be inserted asceptically at the bedside or in the operating room
  • Inserted usually over the nondominant posterior frontal lobe
  • Tip of catheter should be in the lateral ventricle

From: *Current Clinical Neurology: Handbook of Neurocritical Care*
Edited by: A. Bhardwaj, M. A. Mirski, J. A. Ulatowski © Humana Press Inc., Totowa, NJ

- Cannot be placed if ventricles are collapsed
- Can be used for controlled CSF drainage
- Integrity of the closed drainage/monitoring system should be maintained
- Can be zeroed to the external auditory meatus as "reference"
- Infection rate up to 27% and increases significantly after 5 d
- Prophylactic antibiotics against skin flora are recommended
  □ Oxacillin 1 g IV q 6 h
  □ Clindamycin 600 mg IV Q 8 h
  □ Ancef 1 g IV Q8 h
- Subarachnoid Bolt:
  - Can be placed over either hemisphere
  - Cannot be used for CSF drainage
  - May give false reading because of intracranial pressure gradients
  - Utilized when ventricles are collapsed as a result of global brain swelling
  - Incidence of infection is very low. Prophylactic antibiotics are not recommended
  - Dampening of waveform may occur as a result of collection of debris in the system
- ◆ Solid state devices:
  - Do not require fluid coupling for pressure transduction
  - Less prone to waveform dampening and artifacts from poor coupling
  - Cannot be zeroed once it has been inserted
  - Can be placed in the ventricles, brain parenchyma, subdural space
  - Significant drift may occur after 5 d
  - Low rate of infection
  - Expensive because they require a separate module to interface with intensive care unit (ICU) monitoring system for recording

Cerebral Edema and Elevated Intracranial Pressure: Fundamental Principles

◆ Cerebral edema (increased brain-water content) and elevated intracranial pressure (ICP) are frequently encountered in clinical practice in patients with brain injury from diverse etiologies including:
  - Traumatic brain injury
  - Cerebral ischemia

- Neoplastic disease
- Intracerebral hemorrhage
- Fulminant Hepatic failure
- Meningitis or encephalitis

♦ Global increases in ICP may compromise cerebral perfusion pressure (CPP) (mean arterial blood pressure [MAP]-ICP) and cerebral blood flow (CBF) leading to cerebral ischemia and irreversible brain injury

♦ Focal cerebral edema may or may not translate into elevated ICP

♦ Focal cerebral edema can act as a mass that may lead to:
  - Lethal intracranial compartmental shifts causing compression of vital brain structures characterized with a constellation of symptoms and signs (herniation syndromes) (*see* Table 1)
  - Herniation syndromes can exist in the face of normal global ICP

♦ Traditionally cerebral edema has been classified
  - Cytotoxic edema:
    • As a consequence of cellular energy failure (Na^+–K^+ pump disruption)
    • Involves the gray and white matter
    • Predominantly intracellular
    • Blood–brain barrier is intact
    • Occurs in ischemic/hypoxic brain injury, water intoxication, Reye's syndrome
  - Vasogenic edema:
    • Secondary to increased vascular permeability to plasma components because of dysfunction of glial foot processes
    • Predominantly extracellular
    • Involves the white matter predominantly
    • Due to increased vascular permeability to plasma components
    • Blood–brain barrier is disrupted
    • Occurs with tumor, inflammation (meningitis, abscess), intracranial hemorrhage (ICH),
    • Sensitive to steroids
  - Hydrocephalic edema:
    • Secondary to obstruction of CSF pathways leading to its periventricular extravasation
    • Predominantly extracellular
    • Involves the white matter predominantly
    • Blood–brain barrier is intact
    • Occurs with hydrocephalus

Table 1
Types of Herniation Syndromes[a]

Syndrome	Clinical manifestations
Subfalcian or Cingulate	Usually a diagnosis made on neuroimaging studies (CT, MRI)
	Cingulate gyrus herniates under the falx cerebrii (anterior much more common than posterior)
	Can lead to compression of ACA resulting in infarction manifesting as contralateral lower extremity paraesis
Central Tentorial	Caused by downward displacement of one or both cerebral hemispheres causing compression of diencephalon and midbrain through tentorial notch
	Usually a result of centrally located space occupying lesions (tumors, hematoma)
	Leads to impaired consciousness and eye movements
	ICP is elevated
	Manifests as bilateral decorticate or decerebrate posturing
Lateral Transtentorial (Uncal)	Most common herniation syndrome seen in clinical practice
	Usually a result of laterally located masses (tumors, hematomas)
	Medial part of temporal lobe (uncus and parahippocampal gyrus) is displaced and forced into the oval-shaped tentorial opening (incisura) at the level of midbrain
	Injury to the outer fibers of the occulomotor nerve, ipsilateral pupillary dilatation (Hutchinson pupil) and ptosis. Compression of midbrain and PCA resulting in depressed level of consciousness, contralateral hemiparesis, decerebrate posturing, central neurogenic hyperventilation
	ICP is elevated
	Unilateral or bilateral infarctions of the occipital lobe because of compression of PCA
	May lead to obstructive hydrocephalus resulting from aqueductal and perimesencephalic cisternal compression
	Lateral flattening of midbrain, zones of necrosis, and secondary hemorrhages in tegmentum, base of subthalamus, midbrain, and upper pons ("Duret" hemorrhages)
Cerebellar–Foramen Magnum	Downward mesial displacement of cerebellar hemispheres (ventral parafolliculi or tonsillae) though foramen magnum leading to medullary compression episodic tonic extension ("cerebellar fits"), arching of the back and neck, extension and internal rotation of limbs, loss of consciousness, cardiac arrhythmias, precipitous changes in BP, heart rate, small pupils, ataxic breathing, disturbance of conjugate gaze and quadriparesis
	May be unilateral or bilateral
	Respiratory arrest is the most fatal manifestation
	Most frequently caused by masses in the posterior fossa

(continued)

Table 1 *(continued)*

Syndrome	Clinical manifestations
External	A result of penetrating injuries to the skull (e.g., gunshot wound or skull fractures)
	ICP may not be elevated due to dural opening and loss of intracranial contents (CSF and brain tissue)
Upward	Not common
	Usually iatrogenic following placement of IVC for external CSF drainage in the presence of a posterior fossa mass lesion

[a]Prompt recognition is paramount toward instituting resuscitative therapies.
Abbr: ACA, anterior cerebral artery; PCA, posterior cerebral artery.
Modified from Harukuni et al., 2002.

- Hydrostatic edema:
  - A result of elevated systemic blood pressure
  - Involves gray and white matter
  - Is predominantly extracellular
  - Blood–brain barrier is disrupted
- Osmotic edema:
  - A result of plasma hypo-osmolality
  - Involves the gray and white matter
  - BBB is intact
  - Is intracellular and extracellular
  - Causes include syndrome of inappropriate secretion of anti-diuretic hormone (SIADH) and overhydration

Treatment of Cerebral Edema and Elevated Intracranial Pressure

♦ From a therapeutic perspective there is considerable overlap in the management of cerebral edema with or without elevated ICP
- General:
  - Avoid shivering, agitation, or fever
  - Maintenance of euvolemic or slightly hypervolemic state
  - Pressors as needed to maintain CPP (usually >70 mmHg)
  - Facilitate venous outflow (head elevation to 30° and midline position)
- Specific:
  - Controlled hyperventilation ($PaCO_2$ 25–30 mmHg)
  - External CSF drainage
  - Osmotic therapy (osmotic agents, diuretics)
  - Metabolic suppression (barbiturates, propofol)

- Blood–brain barrier integrity (Steroids)
- Decompressive surgery
- Hypothermia

Osmotic Agents

♦ Their use remains the cornerstone of medical therapy for cerebral edema and elevated ICP

♦ An ideal osmotic agent should have the following properties:
  - Is not actively metabolized
  - Is nontoxic
  - Predominantly remains in the intravascular compartment to cause egress of water from the brain
  - Few side effects

♦ Urea:
  - Introduced into clinical practice in the 1940s
  - Is not used presently because it is actively metabolized
  - Causes vein irritation
  - Approximately 40% crosses the blood–brain barrier

♦ Mannitol:
  - Been in clinical use since 1960s and remains the standard agent of choice
  - Simple alcohol derivative of sugar mannose
  - Stable in solution
  - Approximately 90% is retained in the intravascular compartment
  - Has nonosmotic properties:
    - Enhances cerebral blood flow (CBF) and oxygen delivery
    - Free radical scavenger
    - Decreases CSF production and enhances CSF reabsorption

♦ Glycerol:
  - More commonly used in continental Europe (out of tradition)
  - Naturally occurring in mammalian tissues
  - Decrease ICP when given orally without significant gastrointestinal side effects
  - May produce hemolysis when given rapidly intravenously
  - Approximately 50% crosses the blood–brain barrier
  - Use of glycerol in the United States has become almost negligible

♦ Hypertonic saline solutions:
  - Oldest osmotic agents historically
  - Completely excluded from blood–brain barrier

– Have been used for small volume resuscitation in shock
– Improves physiological parameters (e.g., systemic blood pressure [BP], cardiac index, and tissue perfusion)
– Enhances cerebral blood flow (CBF) and oxygen delivery
– Several clinical studies have demonstrated their efficacy in treatment of cerebral edema and elevated ICP

Therapeutic Rationale and Goals of Osmotherapy

♦ In normal individuals, the serum osmolality (270–290 mOsm/L) is relatively constant
♦ Serum sodium (Na^+) concentration is an estimate of body water osmolality
♦ Under ideal circumstances, serum osmolality can be calculated from the formula:
♦ Serum Osmolality (mOsm/L) = $2[Na^+ + K^+$ (meq/L)] + [plasma glucose (mg/dL)]/18 + [BUN (mg/d/L)]/2.8
♦ Since urea is freely diffusible across cell membranes, blood urea nitrogen (BUN) is less important and serum sodium and plasma glucose are the key elements in altering serum osmolality
♦ The goal of osmotherapy for cerebral edema associated with brain injury is to maintain a euvolemic or a slightly hypervolemic state
♦ A hyposmolar state should always be avoided in any patient with an acute brain injury
♦ A serum osmolality in the range of 300–320 mOsm/L is recommended for patients with acute brain injury who demonstrate poor intracranial compliance

Osmotherapy Protocol for Cerebral Resuscitation (*see* Fig. 1)

Potential Complications of Osmotic Agents

♦ Mannitol:
– Dehydration secondary to free water diuresis. Can be insidious and lead to hypernatremia
– Hypotension is usually transient especially during rapid infusions and in patients that are volume depleted
– Hemolysis owing to rapid osmotic shifts across red cell membranes
– Hyperkalemia due to renal insufficiency as a consequence of volume depletion
– Renal insufficiency due to volume depletion

ACUTE BRAIN INJURY

↓

GCS ≤ 8
Cerebral edema or compartmental shits on head CT scan
Compression of vital brain structures

↓

Tracheal intubation and mechanical ventilation
ICP monitoring
CSF Drainage if feasible

↓

Monitor GCS; Serial neurological examinations
Maintain normovolemia or slight hypervolemia
Keep CPP > 70 mmHg (with vasopressors if needed)
Maintenance fluids – 0.9%, 2% or 3% saline
Monitor serum Na+ Q 4-6 H with goals >140 mEq/L
Osmotic diuretics

↓

Signs of clinical herniation
ICP > 20 mmHg

↓

Hyperventilation to keep $PaCO_2$ 25-30 mmHg
Osmotic diuretics- Furosemide
Maintain normovolemia, CPP > 70 mmHg
Mannitol 0.5-1.0 g/Kg IV bolus; Serum osmolality goals 300-320 mOsm/L
Maintain iv fluids 2%-3% saline; Maintain serum Na+ 145-155 mEq/L
23.4% saline IV bolus for refractory intracranial hypertension
Pharmacologic coma with barbiturates (? Propofol)
Consider surgical decompression (decompressive hemicraniectomy, lobectomy)

Fig. 1. Suggested algorithm for cerebral resuscitation following traumatic brain injury that can be extrapolated to other brain injury paradigms. (Adapted from Bhardwaj and Ulatowski; 2000 and Harukuni et al.; 2002.)

- Congestive heart failure and pulmonary edema owing to rapid expansion of plasma volume, usually in patients with compromised renal function
- Rebound cerebral edema due to reversal of osmotic gradient between the blood and the brain in areas of compromised blood–brain barrier

♦ Hypertonic saline (HS) has a better side effect profile than mannitol. There have been no phase I trials to date. Theoretical concerns include:

- Myelinolysis (especially with rapid over-correction of preexisting hyponatremia)
- Encephalopathy (confusion), lethargy, seizures, occasionally coma
- Pulmonary edema, heart failure (especially in patients with poor cardiovascular reserve)
- Hypotension (paradoxical response to rapid intravenous bolus injections)
- Coagulopathy (prolonged activated prothrombin and partial thromboplastin times and decrease in platelet aggregation)
- Phlebitis (concentrated solutions are given through the peripheral route); central venous route of administration is recommended
- Subdural hematomas or effusions may occur as a result of shearing of bridging veins as a result of hyperosmolar contracture of the brain away from the dura
- Electrolyte disturbances (e.g., hypokalema). May lead to cardiac arrhythmias
- Hyperchloremic academia, hence, use of HS solutions as a mixture of chloride:acetate (50:50) is recommended
- Rapid withdrawal of therapy with HS may result in rebound cerebral edema, leading to elevated ICP or herniation syndromes

Key Points

♦ Cerebral edema and elevated ICP may cause secondary brain injury from compromised CBF
♦ Osmotic agents constitute the cornerstone of medical therapy for cerebral edema and elevated ICP
♦ Mannitol is the most widely used osmotic agent
♦ Hypertonic saline solutions may prove to be superior to mannitol, although no randomized controlled trials have been performed to date.

Suggested Reading

Harukuni I, Kirsch JR, and Bhardwaj A. Cerebral resuscitation: role of Osmotherapy. *J Anesthesia* 2002;16:229–237.

Bhardwaj A and Ulatowski JA. Cerebral edema: hypertonic saline solutions. _Curr Treat Opt Neurol_ 1999;1:179–187.

Bingaman WE and Frank JI. Malignant cerebral edema and intracranial hypertension. _Neurol Clin_ 1995;3:479–509.

Klatzo I. Neuropathological aspects of cerebral edema (1967). _J Neuropathol Exp Neurol_ 1967;26:1–14.

Paczynski RP. Osmotherapy:basic concepts and controversies. _Crit Care Clin_ 1997;13:105–129.

Zornow MH. Hypertonic saline as a safe and efficacious treatment of intracranial hypertension. _J Neurosurg Anesth_ 1996;8:175–177.

Qureshi AI, Suarez JI, Bhardwaj A, et al. Use of hypertonic (3%) saline/acetate infusion in the treatment of cerebral edema: effect on intracranial pressure and lateral displacement of the brain. _Crit Care Med_ 1998;26:440–446.

Suarez JI, Qureshi AI, Bhardwaj A, et al. Treatment of refractory intracranial hypertension with 23.4% saline. _Crit Care Med_ 1998;26:1118–1122.

Simma B, Burger R, Falk M, Sacher P, and Fanconi S. A prospective, randomized, and controlled study of fluid management in children with severe head injury: lactated Ringer's solution versus hypertonic saline. _Crit Care Med_ 1998;26:1265–1270.

Schwarz S, Georgiadis D, Aschoff A, and Schwab S. Effects of hypertonic (10%) saline in patients with raised intracranial pressure after stroke. _Stroke_ 2002;33:136–40.

6 Traumatic Brain Injury

Romergryko G. Geocadin

Epidemiology

♦ Traumatic brain injury (TBI) is a leading cause of disability and death among children and young adults in the US
♦ Of the estimated 1.5 million persons who sustain TBI annually, about 230,000 persons are hospitalized and survive, 50,000 die, and up to 90,000 will have long-term disability
♦ The risk of TBI is highest among adolescents, young adults, and the elderly (>75 yr old)
♦ Among the most common causes of TBI:
 – Motor vehicle crashes are the leading cause for TBI hospitalization
 – Violence (suicide and assault) is the leading cause of TBI deaths
 – Falls are the leading cause of TBI in the elderly

Pathophysiology

♦ Mechanical forces are responsible for traumatic brain injury Common factors leading to injury are:
 – Direct or contact injury
 – Acceleration and deceleration forces
 – Rotational (torsional) forces
♦ TBI caused by these forces are divided into:
 –Primary brain injury resulting from direct tissue damage at time of injury (*see* Table 1)
 – Secondary brain injuries, that are the common complications related to the primary injury (*see* Table 2)

From: *Current Clinical Neurology: Handbook of Neurocritical Care*
Edited by: A. Bhardwaj, M. A. Mirski, J. A. Ulatowski © Humana Press Inc., Totowa, NJ

Table 1
Primary Brain Injury

Diffuse injury	*Focal injury*
Diffuse axonal injury	Vascular injury
Diffuse vascular injury	Epidural hemorrhage
	Subural hemorrhage
	Subarachnoid hemorrhage
	Intracerebral hemorrhage
	Intraventricular hemorrhage
	Axonal injury
	Contusional injury
	Laceration

Table 2
Secondary Brain Injury

Diffuse and focal hypoxic–ischemic injury
Diffuse and focal brain edema
Intracranail hypertension
Hydrocephalus
Infection

Primary Brain Injury—Diffuse Injury

♦ Diffuse axonal injury (DAI):
 – Diffuse damage to axons (total or partial disruption of transport and impulse conduction) in the cerebral hemispheres, corpus callosum, brain stem, and cerebellum
 – Usually with acceleration–deceleration injury. Sometimes in direct contact injury
 – Broad spectrum of clinical presentation
 • Mild cases have brief unresponsiveness, confusion, and amnesia with some residual neurological dysfunction
 • Severe cases with loss of consciousness for days to weeks or, with persistent vegetative state. Residual neurological dysfunction is typical
 • Head computed tomography (CT)—may initially be normal. Diffuse edema may be noted with obliteration of the cerebrospinal fluid (CSF) cisterns and midline shift. May be associated with focal hemorrhages

– Diffuse vascular injury (DVI) :
  • Diffuse small multiple hemorrhages throughout the brain
  • Similar causes as DAI
  • May present similarly as DAI but is associated with higher mortality than DAI
  • Head CT—multiple hemorrhages throughout the brain

Primary Brain Injury—Focal Injury

♦ Vascular injuries (*see* Table 3)
♦ Focal axonal injury:
  – Localized damage to axons (total or partial disruption of transport and impulse conduction)
  – May present with focal neurologic deficit depending on site of injury
♦ Contusional injury:
  – Focal injury from localized mechanical forces that damage small blood vessels and brain parenchyma
  – Focal bleeding is hallmark
  – May range from microhemorrhages but may become confluent and cause mass effect
  – Commonly caused by acceleration–deceleration injury that impact on bony prominence of the skull (temporal, frontal, and occipital areas)
  – Common types of contusion include:
    • Coup contusion: direct injury at the site of impact
    • Contrecoup: injury at the site opposite to the site of impact
♦ Laceration:
  – Primary disruption of neural parenchyma at time of injury
  – Typically on the surface. Gray matter but can extend to the white matter
  – Commonly seen with penetrating head injuries
  – Types of laceration are:
    • Direct laceration: caused by foreign body (missile) or overlying fractured skull
    • Indirect laceration: caused by tissue deformation as a result of mechanical forces, common in temporal or inferior frontal lobe
♦ In cases of mild head injury, a concussive syndrome may occur:
  – Concussion is the brief alteration in consciousness with neurologic dysfunction such as amnesia, confusion, disorientation,

impaired memory, delayed or impaired verbal and motor responses, and incoordination
- Loss of consciousness, such as unresponsiveness to stimuli or brief coma-like states, may occur but is not necessary for the diagnosis
- Generally, there are no gross or microscopic abnormalities associated. CT scan and magnetic resonance imaging (MRI) show no or minimal abnormalities
- Post-concussive syndrome may occur after mild head injury. Associated problems include: difficulty with concentration, hyperacusis, vertigo, and personality changes

Physical Examination

The Glasgow Coma Scale (GCS) is a tool used widely to assess neurological traumatic brain injury. The GCS is scored based on eye, verbal and motor responses (*see* Table 3).

In patients with head trauma, the initial GCS is used to stratify the severity:
- Mild injury with GCS 14–15
- Moderate injury with GCS 9–13
- Severe injury with GCS 3–8

The detail and extent of general and neurological examination is usually dictated by the severity of initial clinical presentation. It is therefore important to individualize examination.

General Survey of Head Trauma Patients

♦ Visualization of cranium:
  - Evidence of base of the skull fracture:
    • Battle sign: retro-auricular ecchymosis
    • Racoon's eyes: peri-orbital ecchymosis
    • CSF otorrhea
    • CSF rhinorrhea
    • Hemotympanum
  - Evidence of facial fracture:
    • Lefort fracture (stability of facial bones and zygoma)
    • Orbital rim fracture (with step-off abnormality)
  - Proptosis and periorbital edema
♦ Extracranial vascular injury:
  - Evidence for traumatic carotid dissection (presence of pulse and auscultation for bruits). Horners syndrome may be observed

- Evidence for traumatic carotid cavernous fistula (eye globe auscultation for bruit)
◆ Evidence for associated spine trauma (evaluate cervical to sacral spine)
◆ Evaluate nonneurological trauma:
   - Chest
   - Abdomen
   - Pelvis
   - Evaluation of extremities

Focused Neurological Examination in Head Trauma Patients

◆ Mental status evaluations:
   - Document level of consciousness and cognitive function
   - Serial evaluation may signal deterioration
◆ Cranial nerves (CN):
   - Olfactory nerve: avulsion of CN 1 may lead to anosmia, but is difficult to assess acutely
   - Optic nerve:
      • In a conscious patient, ask the patient for the best visual response. Test each eye separately
      • Evaluate best visual performance using a vision card or reading a newspaper. If abnormal, proceed with counting fingers, color identification, or detection of hand motion or light
      • If patient is unconscious, check for afferent pupillary response. This may indicate an optic nerve injury
      • Fundoscopic examination may be helpful in documenting papilledema, retinal hemorrhage, or detachment
   - CN 3: Evaluate pupillary light response:
      • Absence of pupillary light reflex in a dilated pupil may signify uncal herniation
   - CN 3, 4, and 6: impaired extraocular movement may suggest injury to parts of these cranial nerves
   - CN 7: direct injury to peripheral nerve will lead to paralysis of the upper and lower facial muscles on the affected side.
   - CN 8: unilateral hearing loss may result from injury to the temporal bone (middle ear dysfunction)
   - CN 9, 10, 11, and 12: involvement of these cranial nerves may suggest injury to the lower brainstem or parts of the CN as it exits the base of the skull

Table 3
Focal Traumatic Vascular Injury

Types by location	Common causes	Clinical presentation	Diagnostic work-up	Management
Epidural hematoma	Head trauma, associated with skull fracture with laceration of the middle meningeal artery. Also seen in nontraumatic conditions such as coagulopathies and vascular malformation.	Biphasic with rapid progression ("lucid" Interval) Initial loss of consciousness (resulting from concussion) followed by lucidity then coma (resulting from hematoma expansion, increased ICP and herniation)	Head CT scan finding: Hyperdense, convex lucency that usually respects skull suture lines. Skull fracture may be seen on bone window.	Emergent surgical evacuation
Subdural hematoma	Head trauma from severe to mild, sometimes not apparent with avulsion of the bridging veins. Common in the elderly, neonates and infants. Also seen in nontraumatic conditions such as coagulopathies and vascular malformation	Usually slow but can be rapid. Initial presentation can be nonspecific such as behavioral changes with decreasing level of consciousness to weakness and coma.	Head CT scan findings: Acute (<1 wk): Hyperdense, concave fluid collection in the subdural space. Subacute (1–3 wk): Isodense concave fluid collection. A subdural window CT may help define the clot. Chronic: (>3 wk): Hypodense concave fluid collection.	Surgical evacuation

Subarachnoid hemorrhage	Head trauma is most common cause but accular saneurysmal rupture is also a common cause. Occasionally this can be caused by arteriovenous malformations.	Sudden onset of severe headache with abrupt or gradual loss of consciousness. Focal neurological findings with cranial nerve and motor deficit may be noted.	Head CT scan findings: Hyperdense lucency in the subarachnoid space, especially in the basal cisterns, usually with associated increase in ventricular size. Cerebral angiography is needed to define the aneurysm or malformation	Aneurysmal clipping by surgery or endovascular coiling
Intra-parenchymal hemorrhage	Hypertension is a common cause for the primary bleeds. Secondary causes, such as trauma, coagulopathy account for majority of the cases.	Clinical manifestation is dependent on the site and size of the hematoma. Reduction of consciousness is common in large clots with high intracranial pressure and brainstem compression. Cortical involvement may cause focal motor, sensory and language deficit. Brainstem involvement will lead to cranial nerve and arousal problems. Coordination is altered with cerebellar lesion.	Head CT scan finding: Hyperdense lucency most common at the basal ganglia, thalamus, brainstem (pons) cerebellum and cortex. Cerebral angiogram and magnetic resonance imaging may be necessary. Traumatic ICH is common in temporal, inferior frontal and occipital areas.	Hematoma evacuation may be a life-saving procedure but provides no definite benefit on functional outcome. Hemicraniectomy is under investigation.
Intra-ventricular hemorrhage (IVH)	Is usually related to hypertension or trauma. May be an extension of bleeding from other sites (such as basal ganglia, thalamus and subarachnoid bleed.	IVH commonly causes reduction in level of consciousness to coma.	Head CT scan finding: Hyperdense lucency in the ventricular system. Hydrocephalus is commonly associated.	External ventricular drain for drainage of CSF and blood.

♦ Motor examination:
  – In cooperative patients, evaluate power and range of motion
  – In uncooperative patients, assess the motor response to noxious stimuli. Carefully differentiate purposeful movements from posturing, or stereotypical responses
  – Evaluation of movement for right–left symmetry
♦ Sensory examination:
  – In a cooperative patient, assessment to pinprick in all major dermatomes on the trunk and extremities (to assess the ventral spinal cord function). It is also important to assess the dorsal cord functions by joint position sense
  – In uncooperative patients, keen observation is important. Application of noxious stimulation to areas above and below the cervical cord may help rule out significant cervical cord injury. Facial responses such as grimace or vocalization are noted along with the description of responses in the extremities
♦ Reflexes:
  – Abnormality of deep tendon reflexes (DTRs) may suggest presence of spinal cord, root or nerve injury. Asymmetry of DTRs will suggest the location of the injury
  – Reflexes suggestive of cortico-spinal injury such as Babinski sign and the Hoffman sign may be helpful in localizing the lesion
  – In cases of suspected spinal cord injury, assessment of the rectal tone, anal wink and bulbocavernous reflex are helpful

Diagnostic and Therapeutic Management of Head Trauma

♦ The Brain Trauma Foundation (BTF) guidelines for the management of head trauma are incorporated in the approach to the care of head trauma patients
♦ The BTF recommendations are made at three levels as:
  – Standards based primarily on scientific data
  – Guidelines based on some scientific data but insufficient to a standard of care
  – Options are suggestions by the foundation based on little scientific evidence
The main goals in the diagnostic and therapeutic management are:
  – Correction of the primary pathology
  – Prevention and correction of secondary injury
  – Promotion of normal electrical function of the brain

♦ Critical care approach:
  – The overall approach to a critically ill patient is similar for head trauma patients, namely A, airway; B, breathing; C, circulation–(leading to clinical stabilization that allows to safely perform); D, diagnostics. A figure outlining the initial management of patients with severe head injury is provided in Fig. 1
♦ Airway breathing and circulation:
  – The BTF's recommendation does not reach a standard but provides the following Guidelines: hypotension (systolic blood pressure [SBP] <90 mmHg) and hypoxia (with oxygen saturation <90% or PaO_2 <60 mmHg) must be monitored, avoided or immediately corrected
  Option: to keep the SBP >90 mmHg with fluid and cerebral perfusion pressure (CPP) >70 mmHg. In patients with GCS <9, who are not able to maintain good oxygenation, supplemental oxygen may be provided. This may require endotracheal intubation and mechanical ventilatory support
  –Neurological deterioration has been noted when CPP is low. CPP is the difference of the mean arterial pressure (MAP) and the intracranial pressure (ICP)
  – It is important to note that both hypoxia and ischemia will not only cause a direct neuronal injury but also increase the likelihood of ICP elevation because of the vasodilatory response

Initial Management: Sedation and Neuromuscular Blockade

♦ No outcome studies are available addressing sedation of patients with severe head injury
♦ Intensive care unit (ICU) stay may be prolonged with routine sedation and neuromuscular blockade
♦ Neurologic assessment may be impaired
♦ The decision to sedate patients needs to be individualized, such as agitation during transport, with evidence of ICP elevation, difficulty with mechanical respiratory support
♦ Agents commonly used for sedation include: Propofol, short acting benzodiazepine (i.e., midazolam). Fentanyl, as an analgesic can also be used for sedation and provides pain relief after traumatic injury

INITIAL MANAGEMENT

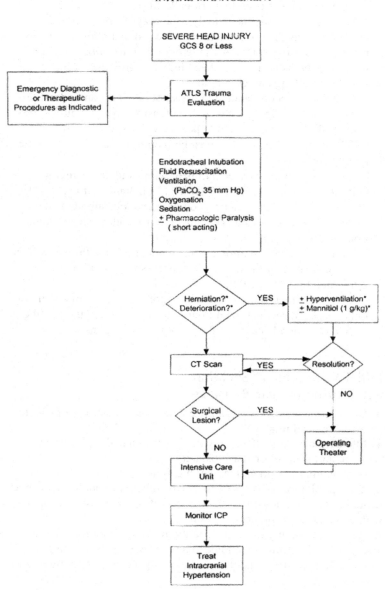

Diagnostic Components: Includes Diagnostic Imaging and ICP Monitoring.

♦ Head CT scan (unenhanced) is the test of choice for patients who have moderate- to high-risk of injury after head trauma as CT scan reveals hemorrhage and bony injury

♦ Indication for head CT include: GCS ≤14, progressive headache, decline in level of consciousness, alcohol or drug intoxication, seizure, unreliable history, vomiting, amnesia, signs of skull fracture, facial injury, penetrating skull injury, suspected child abuse or focal or abnormal neurological finding

♦ About 90% of patients with significant head injury have abnormal initial head CT

♦ Outcome of patients with normal head CT on admission is largely dependent on extracranial injuries and complications

♦ Absence of abnormalities on CT on admission does not rule out ICP elevation

♦ A skull x-ray (SXR) is only helpful if CT scan is not available. SXR may show fractures or penetrating injury. But in generally SXR is not recommended in addition to CT

♦ Spine fracture is identified early. Spinal injury precaution is necessary until spine fracture is determined (*see* Chapter 12)

ICP Monitoring

♦ The need for ICP monitoring is provided in the BTF guidelines in those patients with high likelihood of significant ICP elevation. The detection ICP elevation will lead to prompt therapy, thereby potentially preventing further injury

♦ Patients that require ICP monitoring are the following:
  – Severe head injury with GCS 3–8 with either:
    • Abnormal CT scan on admission
    • Normal CT scan with 2 or more: age >40, motor posturing, SBP <90 mmHg

♦ ICP monitoring is not routinely indicated in patients with mild to moderate head injury

♦ ICP monitoring may be undertaken in conscious patients with traumatic mass lesion

---

Fig. 1. *(previous page)* BTF guidelines for initial management of patients with severe TBI. From J Neurotrauma 2000;17(6–7):463–469, with permission.

♦ The recommendations for ICP monitoring system are:
  – ICP monitored by intraventricular catheter connected to an
  external strain gauge is preferred
  – Most accurate, low cost, and reliable
  – Allows for therapeutic CSF drainage
♦ Parenchymal ICP monitoring with fiberoptic or strain gage
catheter tip transduction is adequate for ICP monitoring but has the
potential for a measurement drift
♦ Subarachnoid ICP (bolts) monitors are less accurate but are an
option especially when the ventricle is not accessible because of
edema or mass effect
♦ Once ICP monitoring is undertaken, the BTF provide the follow-
ing guidelines for the initiation of treatment:
  – Sustained ICP elevation ≥20–25 mmHg
  – ICP treatment should be corroborated with clinical exam and
  CPP data
  – Prolonged ICP elevation >25mmHg is associated with neuro-
  logic deterioration

Medical Treatment of ICP Elevation

♦ Hyperventilation (HV) causes vasoconstriction leading to attenuation in ICP elevation:
  – The BTF provides as a standard that in the absence of ICP elevation, prolonged HV ($PaCO_2$ <25 mmHg) should be avoided.
  – As a guideline, prophylactic HV ($PaCO_2$ <35 mmHg) during
  the first 24 h after severe head injury is avoided because it can be
  harmful
  – As an option the BTF provides that:
    • HV may be necessary to reduce ICP elevation for brief peri-
    ods when there is a neurological deterioration
    • HV may be used longer if ICP elevation is refractory to
    sedation, paralysis, CSF drainage, and osmotic therapy
♦ Mannitol has been successfully used to reduce ICP after head
trauma
♦ The BTF guidelines suggest mannitol as a bolus dose of
0.25–1 g/kg IV at the time of ICP elevation or neurological
deterioration
♦ As options, the BTF provides:
  – The use of mannitol prior to ICP monitoring if signs of
  transtentorial herniation are noted or neurological deterioration
  occurs independent of systemic causes

Table 4
Glasgow Coma Score

Best eye response (1–4)
  1 No eye opening
  2 Eye opening to pain
  3 Eye opening to verbal command
  4 Eyes open spontaneously
Best verbal response (1–5)
  1 No verbal response
  2 Incomprehensible sounds
  3 Inappropriate words
  4 Confused
  5 Orientated
Best motor response (1–6)
  1 No motor response
  2 Extension to pain
  3 Flexion to pain
  4 Withdrawal from pain
  5 Localizing pain
  6 Obeys commands

    – With diuresis from mannitol, dehydration must be avoided with fluid replacement
    – Dehydration will lead to hypovolemia and impairment of CPP
    – Serum osmolality is kept <320 mOsm/L to avoid renal injury.
    – Bolus dosing of mannitol is preferred over continuous infusion
♦ Other hyperosmolar therapies such as hypertonic saline (HS) have been used successfully in cohorts of patients after head trauma. The use of these agents has not yet been incorporated in the BTF guidelines. However, current practice includes use of 2–3% NaCl via bolus or continuous IV infusion to raise serum Na^+ to 145–155 mEq/L and following ICP. Stepwise increases in serum Na^+ up to 155 mEq/L may be necessary over several days, but reversal of hypernatremia must be instituted over several days as well to avoid "rebound" cerebral edema and neurologic deterioration. Overall goal is to create an osmotic gradient for egress of water out the brain during peak period of cerebral swelling (approx 2–4 d)

♦ The use of corticosteroids in head trauma is not recommended as a standard by the BTF as there is no consistent reduction in ICP elevation nor improvement in outcome. Complications may be observed, such as infection and gastrointestinal bleeding

♦ The use of barbiturates in cases of hemodynamically stable and salvageable patients with refractory ICP elevation is recommended by the BTF:

   – The recommended barbiturate is pentobarbital with loading dose of 10 mg/kg loading dose over 30 min, then 5 mg/kg every hour for three doses. The maintenance dose is 1 mg/kg/h infusion

   – Barbiturates leads to a reduction in ICP because of the reduction of cerebral blood flow coupled to suppression of brain metabolism

   – Therapy can be guided by the ICP monitor to normalize ICP and by an electroencephalogram (EEG) to show burst suppression activity

   – Barbiturate use is associated with numerous clinical difficulties:

     • Masking of the neurological examination, so an ICP sensor and EEG monitoring will be necessary

     • Requires full ventilatory support

     • Hypotension can be reversed by volume replacement and vasopressors

     • Enteric feeding will be limited by ileus and parenteral nutrition is needed

     • Impaired defenses against infection can be caused by impaired mucociliary action leading to retention of sputum, impaired leucocyte function and the loss of the hypothalamic control for temperature regulation. A mild increase in temperature, a suggestion of an infiltrate in the chest radiograph and other parameters that lead to the suspicion of infection necessitates a thorough investigation for an infection and empiric treatment with broad spectrum antibiotics

Other Medical Management Issues

♦ Use of anti-epileptic drugs (AEDs) after head injury:

   – As a standard, the prophylactic use of AEDs is not recommended for the prevention of late post-traumatic seizures

   – Options for treatment to prevent early post-traumatic seizures. Prevention of early post-traumatic with AEDs in high risk cases such as GCS < 10, cortical contusion, depressed skull fracture, intracerebral hemorrhage (epidural, subdural or parenchymal), penetrating head injury, or observed seizure during the first 24 h

- Prevention of early post-traumatic seizure does not improve overall outcome
♦ Nutritional support of patients after TBI is important:
  - Guidelines provide that 140% resting metabolic expenditure (RME) is replaced in nonparalyzed patients
  - 100% RME replacement is recommended in paralyzed patients
  - Replacement can be done by enteric or parenteral route, with at least 15% calories as protein by d 7
  - Jejunal feeding by gastojejunostomy is the preferred option

Surgical Management

♦ Emergent neurosurgical evaluation is crucial
♦ Placement of intraventricular catheter for both ICP monitoring and therapeutic CSF drainage as indications are determined
♦ Evacuation of acute post-traumatic hematoma can be life saving and can reduce morbidity
♦ Skull and spine fractures need to be detected and corrected as necessary:
  - Common fractures that need surgical intervention:
    • Clinically significant depressed skull fracture
    • Basal skull fracture
    • Craniofacial fracture
    • Spine dislocation

Prognosis and Outcome After Severe Head Trauma

♦ Several parameters in the course of the management of head trauma have been evaluated to help early prognosis:
  - Initial GCS: The probability of poor outcome increases with decreasing GCS:
    • If obtained after adequate resuscitation and without interference from medication, only 20% of patients with GCS = 3 will survive
    • Only 8–10% will have a functional survival (initial GCS = 3)
  - Age at time of trauma: (70% positive prediction value [PPV]).
    • Increasing age, especially >60 yr is a strong independent predictor of poor outcome after head injury
    • Effect of age on outcome was adjusted for systemic complications and intracerebral hematoma

- Pupillary light reflex: the absence of bilateral pupillary light reflex is associated with poor outcome (70% PPV):
  - Direct injury to the globe must be ruled out
  - Must be tested while hemodynamically stable
  - Re-evaluated after evacuation of intracranial hematoma
- Hypotension and hypoxia:
  - Systolic blood pressure of <90 mmHg is associated with poor outcome (67% PPV)
  - Hypotension, combined with hypoxia has higher association with poor outcome (79% PPV)
- Head CT scan:
  - Abnormality on the initial head CT is associated with poor outcome
  - Compressed or absent basal cisterns is associated with increased mortality by 2–3 times.
  - Traumatic subarachnoid hemorrhage is also associated with poor outcome
  - Abbreviated injury score scale and traumatic coma data bank CT classification correlate well with outcome.
  - Midline shift >5 mm in patients >45 yr old is related to poor outcome (78% PPV)
- Extracerebral and intracerebral lesion:
  - Presence of mass lesion leads to poor outcome (78% PPV)
  - Hematoma volume is correlated to outcome
  - Acute subdural hematoma has higher mortality than extradural hematoma

Key Points

♦ Close neurologic monitoring in an ICU setting is standard for patients with severe TBI

♦ Specific therapeutics in patients with TBI include anti-edema and ICP lowering therapies

♦ Surgical evacuation for accompanying space occupying intracranial hematomas may be life-saving in these patients.

♦ Goals for therapy include maintenance of normoxia, normotension, and CPP ≥ 70 mmHg

Suggested Reading

Brain Trauma Foundation (with AANS—Joint section on Neurotrauma and Critical Care). *Management and Prognosis of Severe Traumatic Brain Injury.* Brain Trauma Foundation; 2000.

Reilly R and Bullock R, eds. *Head Injury: Pathophysiology and Management of Severe Closed Head Injury.* Chapman and Hall Medical; 1997.

Greenberg MS. *Handbook of Neurosurgery,* 5th Edition. Thieme Medical Publishers; 2001

Traumatic Brain Injury in the United States: A report to Congress. Centers for Disease Control and Prevention; 1999.

7 Postoperative Care

Robert D. Stevens

Goals of Postneurosurgical Intensive Care

♦ The potentially devastating complications of neurosurgical and neuroendovascular procedures underscore the need for a high level of attentiveness in the postoperative period. The task of postneurosurgical intensive care is to improve surgical outcomes. This involves:
 – Early detection of neurologic deterioration with prompt institution of corrective interventions to avert or limit irreversible injury
 – Restoration of airway, respiratory, hemodynamic, and metabolic function after neurosurgery
 – Prevention, diagnosis, and treatment of nonneurologic complications after neurosurgery

Indications for Postneurosurgical Critical Care Management

♦ Triage should be informed by factors specific to the surgical procedure, anesthetic management, patient, and institution:
 – Procedure:
  • Risk of postoperative neurologic deterioration
   □ Supra- or infratentorial craniotomy
   □ Transphenoidal procedures
   □ Craniofacial surgery
   □ Carotid artery surgery
   □ Major spine surgeries
   □ Neuroendovascular procedures
  • Risk of systemic complications:
   □ Loss of airway (cervical spine surgery, posterior fossa surgery)

From: *Current Clinical Neurology: Handbook of Neurocritical Care*
Edited by: A. Bhardwaj, M. A. Mirski, J. A. Ulatowski © Humana Press Inc., Totowa, NJ

    □ Respiratory failure (posterior fossa, cervical and thoracic spine surgery)

    □ Hemorrhage (spine surgery, cerebrovascular surgery)

– Anesthesia:
- Residual effects of sedative, analgesic, or paralytic agents
- Pharmacologic coma for metabolic suppression (intracranial hypertension)
- Intraoperative hypothermia
- Significant adverse drug reaction (anaphylaxis, malignant hyperthermia)

– Patient:
- Unanticipated intraoperative complication
- Significant coexisting medical/surgical condition:
  - □ Advanced age
  - □ Organ dysfunction: congestive heart failure, coronary artery disease, restrictive or obstructive lung disease, end stage liver or renal disease
  - □ Sepsis
  - □ Trauma
  - □ Coagulopathy

– Institution:
- Presence of a dedicated intensivist/neurointensivist
- Availability of neurosurgery physician coverage
- Presence of a monitored step-down unit
- Nursing staff training and workload:
  - □ In the post-anesthesia care unit
  - □ On the general neurosurgery ward

Epidemiology of Neurosurgical Complications

♦ Complications associated with neurosurgical procedures are listed in Table 1. Perioperative neurosurgical outcomes have consistently improved over the last decades. The following results are from the larger (>100 patients), more recent (since 1990) reports. Rates of nonfatal complications are highly variable, in part reflecting differences in the way complications are defined and reported

♦ Mortality:
- Supratentorial tumor resection: from 1.7 to 5%
- Unruptured intracranial aneurysm surgery: from 0 to 4%
- Ruptured intracranial aneurysm surgery: from 7 to 30%
- Posterior fossa surgery: from 0.3 to 2.5%
- Transphenoidal surgery: from 0 to 2%

- Carotid endarterectomy: from 0.5 to 1%
- Neuroendovascular: from 0.5 to 1%
♦ Nonfatal complications (neurologic and nonneurologic)
  - Supratentorial tumor resection: from 7 to 30%
  - Unruptured intracranial aneurysm surgery: from 12 to 15%
  - Ruptured cerebral aneurysm surgery: from 25 to 70%
  - Posterior fossa surgery: variable depending on pathologic process and location of lesion
  - Transphenoidal surgery: from 8 to 18%
  - Carotid endarterectomy: from 10 to 15%
  - Neuroendovascular: from 5 to 11%
♦ Predictors of postoperative complications:
  - Brain tumor resection: age, infratentorial location, decreased preoperative functional status, emergent admission
  - Unruptured intracranial aneurysm: age, size, posterior circulation location, intraoperative rupture
  - Ruptured intracranial aneurysm: clinical and radiographic grade at presentation
♦ Role of hospital volume:
  - Surgical outcomes after brain tumor resection and cerebral aneurysm surgery are consistently better in centers which manage greater numbers of cases

General Postneurosurgical Management

♦ The initial postoperative evaluation assesses the adequacy of airway, breathing, and circulatory function
♦ The neurologic survey is comprehensive yet emphasizes semiology linked to the surgical procedure:
  - A comparison with preoperative assessments should be made when possible
  - Serial postoperative examinations are invaluable in delineating trends and helping to decide if further tests or procedures are needed
♦ Reports given by neurosurgical and anesthesiology teams may contain critical information:
  - Preoperative neurologic findings not documented elsewhere
  - Intraoperative course:
    • Details of the procedure, surgical complications, neurophysiologic monitoring, preliminary pathology results
    • Limitation of mobility in the postoperative period
    • Anesthesia: Airway, cardiopulmonary management, fluid balance

Table 1
Neurosurgical Complications

Procedure	Complications	
	Neurologic	*Systemic*
Supratentorial tumor resection	Brain edema Stroke Seizure Intracranial hemorrhage Meningitis	Pulmonary infection Urinary tract infection Deep-venous thrombosis Pulmonary embolism
Intracranial aneurysm surgery (unruptured)	Stroke Intracranial hemorrhage Brain edema Seizure Meningitis	Pulmonary infection Urinary tract infection Deep venous thrombosis Pulmonary embolism
Intracranial aneurysm surgery (ruptured)	Stroke Intracranial hemorrhage Vasospasm Hydrocephalus Meningitis	Myocardial injury Neurogenic pulmonary edema Cerebral salt wasting
Arteriovenous malformation exclusion	Edema Intracranial hemorrhage Seizures	Hyperdynamic cardiovascular state
Posterior fossa procedures	Brain edema Brainstem injury Cranial nerve injury Hydrocephalus Intracranial hemorrhage Meningitis	Aspiration Ventilatory failure Hemodynamic instability
Transphenoidal hypophysectomy	Visual field deficit Intracranial hemorrhage Diabetes insipidus CSF leak Meningitis	Panhypopituitarism Hypothyroidism Adrenal Insifficiency
Carotid endarterectomy	Stroke Hyperperfusion syndrome Intracranial hemorrhage Cranial nerve X, XII injury	Myocardial infarction Hypertension Hypotension Neck hematoma
Spine surgery	Epidural hematoma Myelopathy Nerve-root injury Epidural abscess Meningitis	Airway injury/edema Pneumothorax Vascular injury Hemorrhagic shock Ileus
Interventional neuroradiology	Stroke Intracranial hemorrhage	Puncture site: hemorrhage, pseudoaneurysm, arteriovenous fistula Contrast toxicity/ hypersensitivity

– When applicable, rationale for not extubating the patient (*see* "Airway and Respiratory Management")

♦ Pain (*see* Chapter 18):

– Pain after intracranial surgery is often undertreated, out of concern that narcotics will cloud sensorium and induce CO_2 retention. However, poorly controlled pain is associated with significant catecholamine release and increased blood pressure and heart rate, which are undesirable endpoints after craniotomy. In a monitored setting, cautious titration of intravenous fentanyl (25–50 µg) or morphine (1–5 mg) is safe and efficacious

– Surgery of the spine may induce severe postoperative pain and commonly occurs in a context of chronic pain syndromes and narcotic dependence. Aggressive pain management with titration of intravenous narcotics and patient-controlled regimens is recommended

♦ Postoperative nausea and vomiting occur in 30–50% of patients after neurosurgery and can result in hypertension, aspiration, and increased intracranial pressure (ICP). Treatment with intravenous odansetron 4–8 mg, droperidol 0.625–1.25 mg, or metoclopramide 5–10 mg, is indicated. Severe unremitting nausea and vomiting may signal intracranial hypertension

♦ Postoperative shivering occurs in 10% of neurosurgical patients. It is accompanied by a significant increase in oxygen consumption and cardiac output and may be prevented by appropriate intraoperative rewarming. Treatment is with small doses of IV meperidine (15–30 mg). Repeated administration of meperidine is not recommended as it may lead to accumulation of metabolites with proconvulsant effects

♦ Postoperative orders:

– A template for postoperative orders after intracranial surgery is provided in Table 2

– Frequency of clinical assessments should be proportionate to the risk of an acute complication. In most supratentorial tumor resections, this risk decreases exponentially over the first postoperative hours

– Patients should have their head elevated to greater than 30° to facilitate cerebral venous and cerebrospinal fluid drainage and to decrease the risk of nosocomial pneumonia. In patients undergoing evacuation of a chronic subdural hematoma or those who have a significant cerebrospinal fluid (CSF) leak, supine position may be indicated

– Where applicable, it is useful to explicitly state physiologic goals:

Table 2
Template for Postneurosurgical Orders
After Intracranial Surgery

Diagnosis
Procedure
Allergies
Vital signs checks
Neurologic checks
Ventilator parameters
Supplemental oxygen
Nutrition/diet
Activity; head elevation
Physiologic goals

Temperature	(°C)
CPP	(mmHg)
ICP	(mmHg)
MAP	(mmHg)
SBP	(mmHg)
HR	(per min)
CVP	(mmHg)
PAOP	(mmHg)
Urine output	(mL/kg/h)
Fluid balance	(mL/24h)
PaO_2	(mmHg)
$PaCO_2$	(mmHg)
Serum Na	(mmol/L)
Serum glucose	(mmol/L)

Labs (including serum anticonvulsant levels)
Frequent lab checks
EKG
CXR
Intravenous fluids
Anticonvulsants
PRN antihypertensive
PRN pain medication
Thromboembolic prophylaxis
Stress ulcer prophylaxis
Other medications

Abbr: CPP, cerebral perfusion pressure; ICP, intracranial pressure; MAP, mean arterial pressure; SBP, systolic blood pressure; HR, heart rate; CVP, central venous pressure; PAOP, pulmonary artery occlusion pressure.

- Body temperature (emphasize hypothermia after cardiac arrest or avoid hyperthermia after stroke)
- Cerebral perfusion pressure in patients with increased ICP
- Mean arterial pressure in patients with cerebral vasospasm, stroke, or coronary artery disease
- Central venous pressure or pulmonary artery occlusion pressure in patients with cerebral vasospasm
- Systolic blood pressure in patients with/at risk for intracranial hemorrhage
- Heart rate in patients with coronary artery disease
- $PaCO_2$ in patients with decreased intracranial compliance
- Serum Na in patients with diabetes insipidus, secretion of antidiuretic hormone (SIADH), cerebral salt wasting, or those receiving hypertonic saline therapy
- Fluid balance in patients with cerebral vasospasm, renal or cardiac failure
- Urine output in patients with or at risk for diabetes insipidus, cerebral salt wasting, renal insufficiency, or shock

– Anticonvulsants where applicable. Should be dosed to maintain high therapeutic levels

– Prophylaxis against stress ulcers and thromboembolic complications should be systematically prescribed

Neurologic Management

♦ Abnormal neurologic findings are common following intracranial surgery and demand a systematized approach. Several scenarios may be entertained:

– The findings are consistent with the preoperative examination

– The findings are those that would be anticipated from the surgical procedure

– The findings are new and unanticipated (*see* Fig. 1):

- Localizing signs in a patient whose level of consciousness or mental status are altered warrant emergent computerized tomography (CT) imaging and consultation with the neurosurgical team. When focal findings occur in a patient who is alert, it may be reasonable to opt for a period of observation as these may be potentiated by anesthetic effects or neurapraxia from tissue manipulation. Persistence or worsening of signs mandates emergent imaging and neurosurgical consultation

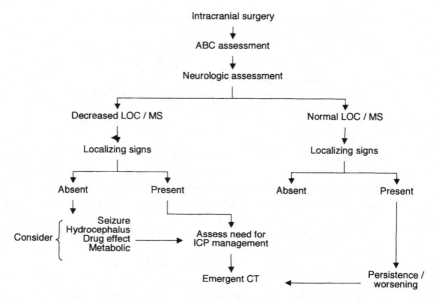

Fig. 1. Neurologic assessment after intracranial surgery.

- Nonlocalizing findings:
  □ Delayed awakening without any element of focality is a diagnostic challenge. In this instance it is useful to consider the different processes that may independently impact on postoperative neurologic function (i.e., effects of surgery, anesthetic agents and other medications, and systemic disturbances [*see* Table 3])

Surgical Complications:

Cerebral Edema (see also Chapter 5)

♦ Manipulation, retraction, and resection of brain tissue induce vasogenic and to a lesser degree cytotoxic edema. Postoperative brain swelling may compound edema associated with tumor, infection, ischemia, or hemorrhage. Surgery for glioblastoma multiforme (GBM), repeat procedures, and lengthy (>6 h) procedures have been linked to a greater risk of swelling and ICP elevation:

  – Focal swelling may lead to compartmental shifts and subfalcine or uncal herniation syndromes or, when less severe, manifest as transient focal neurologic deficits or partial seizures

Table 3
Delayed Awakening After Intracranial Surgery

Brain injury	*Medication*	*Systemic*
Intracranial hemorrhage	Sedatives	Hypothermia
Intraparenchymal	Analgesics	Respiratory
Epidural	Neuromuscular blockers	Hypoxia
Subdural	Anticonvulsants	Hypercapnia
Subarachnoid		Cardiovascular
Stroke		Hypotension
Cerebral edema		Shock
Hydrocephalus		Metabolic/endocrine
Pneumocephalus		Hyponatremia
Seizures		Hypernatremia
Postictal state		Hypoglycemia
Status		Hyperglycemia
Nonconvulsive status		(severe)
		Panhypopituitarism
		Adrenal insufficiency
		Hypothyroidism
		Renal failure
		Hepatic failure
		Sepsis

– Diffuse edema involving both hemispheres typically leads to alterations in mental status and level of arousal; if of sufficient magnitude, increased ICP and central herniation may ensue

– Management of postoperative brain edema is based on the severity of clinical manifestations and on the the underlying pathologic process

• Herniation syndromes require a stepwise approach with control of the airway, short-term hyperventilation, administration of osmotic agents, and ventriculostomy when appropriate. Failure to reverse herniation with these measures should prompt consideration of metabolic suppression with pharmacologic or hypothermic coma, or decompressive craniectomy

• Management of edema with milder clinical repercussions is unclear. Corticosteroids effectively reduce tumor-associated edema but have little effect on postoperative edema. Hypertonic saline solutions have been advocated, but their usefulness in the postneurosurgical setting has not been prospectively evaluated

Intracranial Hemorrhage

♦ Large series indicate between 1.1 and 3% incidence of intracranial hematoma after craniotomy
♦ Risk factors are coagulopathy, emergent surgery, and postoperative hypertension
♦ Clinically significant hemorrhages are most commonly intra-parenchymal (from 43 to 60%) or epidural (from 28 to 33%); in 10–20% of cases, hemorrhage occurrs at a site remote from the surgical procedure
♦ In one study nearly 90% of hemorrhages occurred within 6 h of surgery
♦ Outcomes are markedly worse in patients who develop postoperative intracranial hemorrhage:
  – Between 36 and 55% of patients dead, vegetative or severely disabled at 3 mo
  – Overall mortality 32%
    • Management is controversial, often decided on a case by case basis. There is little data to indicate that surgical evacuation ameliorates outcome

Posterior Fossa Procedures

♦ Edema or hemorrhage are of particular concern given the lesser compliance of this space when compared to the supratentorial compartment. Expanding posterior fossa masses may lead to:
  – Brainstem compression
  – Hydrocephalus
  – Cerebellar displacement through the tentorium (upward herniation) or foramen magnum (tonsillar herniation)

Arteriovenous Malformation (AVM)

♦ Surgical or endovascular management may be complicated by brain swelling or hemorrhage, possibly related to increased perfusion of chronically underperfused peri-lesional blood vessels ("normal pressure breakthrough"). Post-procedure bleeding may also arise from incomplete hemostasis, incomplete resection of the AVM, especially with resection or obstruction of venous outflow

Carotid Endarterectomy

♦ May be complicated by a "hyperperfusion syndrome," in which post-procedure blood flow to the ipsilateral hemisphere increases two- to threefold, leading to edema and hemorrhage and presenting clinically as headache, seizures, or coma

Pneumocephalus

♦ Clinically inconsequential intracranial accumulations of gas are commonly observed after intracranial surgery as well as in the setting of basal skull fractures. Tension pneumocephalus with increased ICP and mass effect may develop, requiring surgical decompression. Conditions promoting tension pneumocephalus include:
  – Aggressive CSF drainage
  – Presence of a ball-valve defect allowing entry but preventing exit of air
  – Intraoperative use of nitrous oxide
  – Rewarming after hypothermia (thermal expansion of air trapped in the cranial vault)

Seizures

♦ Occur in 8 to 18% of untreated patients within 2 wk after undergoing supratentorial craniotomy. Risk decreases with time after surgery, and early postoperative seizures do not predict the later onset of epilepsy:
♦ Risk factors:
  – Preoperative seizure disorder
  – Lesion type: Meningioma, high grade glioma, cerebral abscess, metastatic brain lesions, arteriovenous malformation, and traumatic brain injury
  – Location: greater incidence has been observed with falx and parasagittal meningiomas relative to meningiomas in other sites. Posterior fossa surgery incurs a much lower risk (1.8%)
  – Additional risk factors: low anticonvulsant levels, hypoglycemia, electrolye abnormalities, hypoxemia, acidosis, medications that lower seizure threshold after craniotomy (β-lactam antibiotics)
♦ Seizures may signal postoperative intracranial hemorrhage, edema, stroke, pneumocephalus, or infection. Delayed awakening or changes in mental status after craniotomy may represent nonconvulsive status epilepticus or a prolonged post-ictal state
♦ Seizures increase cerebral metabolic rate ($CMRO_2$), cerebral blood flow (CBF), and intracranial pressure (ICP), and potentially exacerbate edema or hemorrhage. Loss of airway, hypoventilation, and aspiration may induce hypoxia with secondary brain injury

♦ Prophylaxis with phenytoin reduces postoperative seizure incidence by 35 to 50%:

- Addition of perioperative phenytoin in patients who are already receiving anticonvulsants is unlikely to be of benefit. Phenytoin is typically dosed intraoperatively at 15–20 mg/kg IV and continued at 4–6 mg/kg/d. Target serum levels are 15 –20 μg/mL total or 1–2 μg/mL unbound
- Valproic acid is as effective for perioperative prophylaxis as phenytoin with comparable adverse effect rates. It is a reasonable alternative to phenytoin when the latter is contraindicated. Target levels are 50–100 μg/mL. Phenobarbital is another alternative but its prominent sedating effect limits its usefulness

♦ Management of postoperative seizures:

- Assess airway, breathing, and circulatory function
- Lorazepam 1–2 mg iv up to 0.1 mg/kg
- Send serum chemistries, arterial blood gas, phenytoin level.
- Reload with phenytoin 15–20 mg/kg without waiting for levels (target serum level 20–30 μg/mL)
- Emergent CT scan to rule out a precipitating intracranial process
- Consider lumbar puncture if meningitis is a significant risk
- Persistence: initiate status epilepticus protocol (*see* Chapter 15)

Stroke

♦ Postoperative cerebral infarction may occur in a number of neuro-surgical settings:

- Carotid endarterectomy was associated with a 30-d nonfatal stroke incidence of 3%–6% in four large multicentric trials Carotid angioplasty was linked to thromboembolic events in 8.8% of cases
- Unruptured intracranial aneurysms present as ischemic strokes in the vascular territory downstream from the aneurysmal sac in 2–3% of cases. Stroke may occur as a complication of surgical aneurysm repair in 1–5% of cases; this risk is particulatly high with anterior choroidal artery aneurysms (10–20% stroke incidence). Endovascular aneurysm coiling is associated with thromboembolic events in 8.2% of cases
- Ruptured intracranial aneurysms lead to delayed ischemic deficits vasospasm in 30% of cases

– Venous infarction may result from ligation of cortical draining veins or damage to venous sinuses. Excessive retraction or manipulation of sinuses may lead to thrombotic occlusion

– Intracranial hypertension or cerebral herniation may lead to vascular compression and cerebral infarction:

  • Whenever ICP exceeds mean arterial pressure

  • Anterior cerebral artery territory stroke with subfalcine herniation

  • Posterior cerebral artery territory stroke with uncal herniation

– Management options for perioperative stroke are limited. Thrombolytic agents are contraindicated and anticoagulant or antiplatelet agents must be used with caution:

  • Intraoperative burst-suppression with thiopental or propofol may protect cerebral tissue during temporary arterial clipping

  • Acute thrombotic carotid occlusion after endarterectomy requires surgical re-exploration

  • Hyperdynamic therapy and angioplasty may relieve deficits associated with vasospasm

Hydrocephalus

♦ Supratentorial procedures that modify ventricular system anatomy, shunt procedures, posterior fossa procedures, meningitis, and intracranial hemorrhage may lead to acute hydrocephalus. Most common clinical presentation is decreased level of consciousness. Clinical suspicion should be substantiated with emergent CT and drainage options discussed with neurosurgery (*see* Chapter 11)

Pharmacologic Factors

Anesthesia

♦ Cerebral Physiology

♦ General anesthetic agents modify cerebral function by interacting with a number of neuronal receptor sites, and by altering cerebrovascular physiology. Potent inhalational anesthetics (isoflurane, desflurane, sevoflurane, halothane) increase CBF and decrease $CMRO_2$, dissociating neurovascular coupling. In humans halothane increases ICP while the other agents do not. Intravenous anesthetics (e.g., thiopental, propofol, etomidate, midazolam) decrease both CBF and $CMRO_2$ thereby reducing ICP. The weak inhalational agent nitrous oxide and the intravenous agent ketamine increase CBF, $CMRO_2$, and ICP

Excitatory Effects

♦ General anesthetic agents have a predominantly depressant effect on cortical function; however, excitatory phenomena may become apparent during induction and awakening from anesthesia. These include psychomotor agitation, involuntary limb movements, myoclonic jerks, as well as partial and generalized seizures. Enflurane, methohexital, etomidate, and propofol have been linked to perioperative seizures in humans; animal studies indicate that opioids may also trigger seizure activity

Clinical Assessment

♦ General anesthesia may significantly confound neurologic assessment in the early postoperative period. Every aspect of the neurologic examination including level of consciousness, cognition, cranial nerves, motor function, sensory function, cerebellar function, and reflexes may be altered by general anesthesia. Transient neurologic findings in the early postoperative period including nystagmus, clonus, hyperreactive deep tendon reflexes, and Babinski signs, have been linked to residual anesthetic effects. Rapidly resolving focal deficits such as hemiparesis, dysarthria, aphasia, or unilateral pupillary changes may represent underlying brain lesions that are unmasked by anesthesia or sedation. A critical determination is the evolution with time; a declining level of consciousness or worsening deficits are unlikely to be anesthesia-related and mandate emergent imaging (*see* Fig.1)

Pharmacokinetics

♦ Inhalational anesthetics are rapidly eliminated by alveolar ventilation and are unlikely to significantly affect the neurologic examination more than 30 min after administration has ceased
♦ Intravenous anesthetic agents, when administered as a single bolus, have a short duration of action secondary to redistribution. However, repeated doses or infusions (e.g., burst suppression for intraoperative cerebral protection) may lead to accumulation in tissue compartments and a more prolonged effect. This is particularly relevant to thiopental
♦ Elimination kinetics of intravenous anesthetic agents and opioids administered as an infusion may be characterized by the context-sensitive half-time (CSHT), which is the time for the plasma concentration to decrease by 50% after stopping the infusion. CSHT for propofol, remifentanil, and sufentanil at 6 h of infusion are less than

1 h. CSHT for thiopental and fentanyl at 6 h of infusion are significantly longer

Pharmacologic Reversal

♦ Paralytics:
  – Incomplete neuromuscular blockade after anesthesia may induce airway compromise, hypoventilation, anxiety, agitation, hypertension, and tachycardia. Prolonged paralysis after succinylcholine may represent decreased or atypical plasma cholinesterase. Effect of nondepolarizing neuromuscular blockers may be lengthened by hypothermia, acidosis, renal failure, and aminoglycoside antibiotics. Neostigmine 0.05 mg/kg preceded by an anticholinergic agent should be given if there is reasonable uncertainty about residual muscle paralysis
♦ Narcotics:
  – Pupillary constriction, decreased respiratory rate, hypercapnia, decreased alertness, and confusion should prompt consideration of the opioid antagonist naloxone. Naloxone may induce pain, hypertension, tachycardia, and in opioid-dependent individuals acute withdrawal. These effects may be circumvented by judicious titration in 40–80 μg IV increments
♦ Benzodiazepines:
  – Administration of benzodiazepines before or during anesthesia may result in significant delay in emergence. The benzodiazepine antagonist flumazenil is to be used with caution as it may induce seizures and withdrawal
♦ Neurologic effects of other medications used in neurosurgery:
  – Anticonvulsants:
    • Phenytoin toxicity (>20 μg/mL serum level) may present as nystagmus, diplopia, ataxia, asterixis, dysarthria, confusion, and obtundation. Drowsiness is a potential side effect of nearly all anticonvulsants including phenobarbital, clonazepam, valproic acid, carbamazepine, gabapentin, and lamotrigine
    • Corticosteroids, particularly in high doses, may be associated with prominent neuropsychiatric sequelae including agitation, confusion, and psychosis

Airway and Respiratory Management
Respiratory Complications in the Neurosurgical Patient

♦ Respiratory failure is characterized by an inability to achieve adequate oxygenation, ventilation, or both. Pathophysiologic abnor-

malities include alveolar hypoventilation, increased dead-space ventilation, impaired diffusion, ventilation/perfusion mismatch, and arteriovenous shunting:
- Hypoxia correlates with worse outcomes in stroke, traumatic brain injury, and after neurosurgery. When severe it induces cerebral vasodilation and increases ICP
- Hypercapnia promotes cerebral vasodilation and increased ICP

♦ Neurogenic respiratory failure may arise from lesions in the brainstem, spinal cord, peripheral nerves, neuromuscular junction, or muscle. These conditions produce alveolar hypoventilation and, when decompensated, hypercapnia. Management involves treating or stabilizing the underlying pathologic process and providing mechanical ventilatory support

♦ Abnormal breathing patterns:
- Neurogenic hyperventilation syndromes may be observed with intracranial hemorrhage, traumatic brain injury, and pontine lesions
- Cheynes-Stokes consists in alternating hyperpnea and apnea and is seen in extensive bihemispheric injury and congestive heart failure
- Apneustic breathing results from large bilateral pontine lesions, and is characterized by end-inspiratory and end-expiratory pauses
- Ataxic breathing consists in irregularly timed breaths with widely varying tidal volumes and is suggestive of injury to the medulla

♦ Atelectasis is promoted by recumbency and is a frequent complication of surgery and anesthesia. Postoperative lobar or lung collapse may occur secondary to endobronchial intubation or mucus impaction. Atelectasis may worsen gas exchange, increase work of breathing, and promote infection. Preventive strategies include encouraging patients to sit upright, breathe deeply, and cough vigorously. Therapy involves dislodging secretions, recruiting collapsed airways with periodic large tidal volumes, and applying positive end expiratory pressure. Failure of these measures should prompt fiberoptic bronchoscopy

♦ Aspiration. Neurosurgical patients with impaired consciousness and/or bulbar dysfunction are at high risk for aspiration of gastric contents. Severity of lung injury is proportional to the acidity and volume of aspirate. Chemical pneumonitis results if the aspirate is sterile, pneumonia if it contains pathogens. If there is significant risk of further aspiration, tracheal intubation is mandated. Broad spectrum antibiotic coverage is recommended for aspiration pneumonitis that is symptomatic for more than 48 h and for aspiration pneumonia

♦ Pneumonia. Like traumatic brain injury and stroke, neurosurgery is an independent predictor of nosocomial or ventilator-associated pneumonia. Diagnosis is suggested by fever, leukocytosis, radiographic infiltrate, hypoxemia, increased work of breathing, and change in sputum pattern. Antimicrobial therapy should be initially broad, then tapered in accordance with culture data

♦ Pulmonary edema may be hydrostatic, resulting from systolic or diastolic left ventricular failure or fluid overload, or nonhydrostatic, associated with increased pulmonary capillary permeability. The latter category includes acute lung injury and acute respiratory distress syndrome:

– Neurogenic pulmonary edema (NPE) is characterized by a rapidly developing, protein-rich alveolar exsudate that may occur after any neurologic insult but in particular traumatic brain or cord injury, intracranial hemorrhage, and brainstem injury. Presents as a bilateral infiltrates on chest films and increased alveolo-arterial gradient. Pathogenesis may involve transient, sympathetically mediated increase in pulmonary vascular permeability coupled with a decrease in left ventricular compliance. Management consists in:

• Ruling out other causes of pulmonary edema (NPE is a diagnosis of exclusion)

• Identifying and treating, when possible, the underlying neurologic injury

• Supporting oxygenation with mechanical ventilation, supplemental oxygen and PEEP

• Guiding therapy with pulmonary artery catheter or echocardiographic data

– Hemodynamic augmentation therapy for cerebral vasospasm carries an appreciable risk of precipitating pulmonary edema (7 to 17%)

♦ Pulmonary embolism (*see* "Thromboembolism")

Respiratory Support

♦ Oxygen. Based on the principle that hypoxemia aggravates outcome after brain injury, supplemental oxygen should be administered to all neurosurgical in the postoperative period and progressively tapered. Options include nasal prongs (FIO_2 0.24–0.44), Venturi mask (FIO_2 0.24–0.40) and nonrebreather mask (FIO_2 0.40–0.60). In the presence of high-minute ventilation, the delivered FIO_2 may be significantly less. Thus a significantly elevated alveolo-arterial gradient is generally an indication for positive pressure ventilation

♦ Ventilatory support is needed for hypoxemia, hypercapnia, increased work of breathing, and for acute management of intracranial hyperventilation:

– Noninvasive positive pressure ventilation is increasingly recognized as an effective option in managing respiratory failure. It is contraindicated in patients who are comatose, uncooperative, are not protecting their airway, or who are at risk for aspiration. Respiratory failure in these groups mandates endotracheal intubation

– Mechanical ventilation should be individualized according the needs of each patient. Full modes of ventilatory assistance (e.g., assist control ventilation) are needed for patients in the acute phase of hypoxemic hypercapnic respiratory failure and those requiring hyperventilation for intracranial hypertension. Patients with adequate ventilatory function who are intubated for airway protection are adequately managed with minimal support (e.g., CPAP or T-piece)

– PEEP decreases ventilation/perfusion mismatch and intrapulmonary shunting, and is a critically useful adjunct in the management of hypoxemia. PEEP also has significant hemodynamic effects, as it reduces both preload and afterload:

• In the setting of decreased intracranial compliance, high levels of PEEP may be detrimental by reducing cerebral venous outflow. Conversely, abrupt removal of PEEP may be associated with a sudden increase in systemic blood pressure and CPP, promoting cerebral edema in patients with loss of autoregulation

• Clinical studies show that PEEP <10–12 cmH_2O is well tolerated by the vast majority of brain-injured patients

– Hyperventilation induces cerebral vasoconstriction by reducing CBF and CBV. It is an effective intervention for acute increases in ICP. However, in other settings it is controversial:

• Its efficacy beyond 4–6 h declines significantly

• Inappropriate hyperventilation may precipitate cerebral ischemia

• Outcomes after traumatic brain injury may be worsened by chronic hyperventilation

– Recently, a protective ventilatory strategy including low-idal volumes has been shown to improve survival in acute lung injury. This type of ventilation is not appropriate in patients with elevated ICP as it entails a controlled respiratory acidosis, or "permissive hypercapnia"

Discontinuation of Mechanical Ventilation and Extubation

♦ Prompt extubation after neurosurgery is desirable since it facilitates early neurologic assessment, promotes patient comfort, and reduces agitation, hypertension, tachycardia, and increased ICP that may be associated with continued intubation. However, inappropriate extubation may leave the patient vulnerable to respiratory failure, hypoxia, aspiration, hypercarbia, increasing ICP, provoking additional brain injury. Moreover, presence of the endotracheal tube need not impede a thorough neurologic evaluation

♦ In most uncomplicated elective neurosurgery, extubation is performed safely in the operating room or soon thereafter. In more complex situations, decisions regarding extubation must account for interrelated neurologic, pharmacologic, airway, respiratory, hemodynamic, and metabolic factors (*see* Table 4). Accurate knowledge of the surgical procedure will assist in this process:

– Neurologic factors:

• Candidates for postneurosurgical extubation should ideally be able to follow simple commands and not present any new unexplained neurologic abnormality. Decreased level of consciousness is associated with poor airway protection and suggests a pathologic process that may require emergent medical or surgical intervention (*see* Fig. 1 and Table 3).

• Patients with poor and/or worsening intracranial compliance as a result of cerebral edema, tumor, abscess or hemorrhage, with or without raised ICP, should not be extubated

• Patients with repeated seizure activity or in status epilepticus should not be extubated

• Injury to the pons or medulla may alter respiratory center function, leading to central hypo- or hyperventilation syndromes or abnormal respiratory patterns

• Cranial nerves X and IX, and also V, VII, and XII are critical for patency of the airway, physiologic airway protective mechanisms, and swallowing. Dysfunction of these nerves may result from cortical, corticobulbar, brainstem, and direct nerve injury:

□ Posterior fossa surgery (e.g., resection of masses in the region of the 4th ventricle) may induce significant bulbar dysfunction and airway compromise requiring tracheostomy

□ Carotid endarterectomy has been linked to cranial nerves X or XII injury in 4 to 10% of cases. Postoperative cervical edema or hematoma may further compromise airway patency

Table 4
Extubation Checklist After Intracranial Surgery

Neurologic
    No new, unanticipated neurologic abnormality
    No repeated seizures or status
    No intracranial hypertension
    Follows simple commands
    Muscle strength
    No residual narcotic, neuromuscular blocker
    Lower cranial nerve function
        Gag reflex
        Cough reflex
        Tongue protrusion
Airway
    Facial/cervical soft tissue edema
    Cuff-leak test
    Volume of secretions (suctioning q 4 h)
Respiratory
    No increased work of breathing
    Oxygenation
        $PaO2 > 60$ mmHg on 40% $FIO2$
        $PEEP < 10$ mmHg
    Ventilation
        $PaCO2 < 50$ mmHg with spontaneous ventilation
        VE <20 mL/kg
        RR/VT < 100 breaths/min/L
        NIF > -20 cmH_2O
Cardiovascular
    No unresolving shock
    No decompensated congestive heart failure
    No ongoing hemorrhagic process
    No significant dysrhythmia
Metabolic
    Body temperature > 36°C; <38.5°C
    No metabolic acidosis

Abbr: VE, minute ventilation; VT, tidal volume; RR, respiratory rate; NIF, negative inspiratory force.

- High spinal cord injury (above C5) produces partial or total diaphragmatic impairment and ventilatory failure. Injury below C5 decreases expiratory muscle function resulting in decreased cough, mucous impaction and atelectasis

- Critical illness weakness syndromes (acute quadriplegic myopathy, critical illness polyneuropathy) may develop in the setting of prolonged mechanical ventilation, malnutrition, corticosteroids, neuromuscular blockers, sepsis, and multi-organ dysfunction
- Pharmacologic factors:
  - Dosage and timing of agents administered during anesthesia and knowledge of their pharmacokinetic properties are important parameters in the decision to extubate. Residual narcotic or neuromuscular blockade effects may significantly impair airway and ventilatory function and should be compulsively ruled out. If tissues are saturated with a lipophilic narcotic such as fentanyl, reversal with a single dose of naloxone may provide only temporary respiratory adequacy
- Airway factors:
  - In addition to neurogenic airway insufficiency discussed above, the airway may be compromised by edema or hematoma secondary to traumatic intubation, carotid surgery, anterior approaches to cervical spine surgery, protracted prone positioning, massive fluid resuscitation, or in certain allergic reactions. The cuff-leak test is a useful, easily obtainable parameter that can be predictive of successful extubation
  - Copious tracheobonchial secretions requiring frequent suctioning increases the risk of failed extubation, particularly in neurologically compromised patients with weak cough and airway reflexes. Increased secretions may reflect pneumonia, tracheobronchitis, or a noninfectious hypersecretory condition. Purulent secretions and fever in the absence of a pulmonary infiltrate is virtually diagnostic of tracheobronchitis that should be treated with a short course of antibiotics
- Respiratory factors:
  - Candidates for extubation should demonstrate adequacy of oxygenation and ventilation, and should not have evidence of increased work of breathing (accessory muscle use, diaphoresis, anxiety, and tachycardia). Some commonly used respiratory weaning parameters are given in Table 4. These parameters have not been validated in the neurosurgical population
- Hemodynamic factors:
  - Shock, congestive heart failure, myocardial ischemia are associated with unsuccessful weaning and failed extubation

– Metabolic factors:
  • Hypothermia or hyperthermia should be corrected before
  extubation. Conditions associated with increased minute ventilation such as sepsis and metabolic acidosis may significantly
  increase work of breathing and diminish the likelihood of successful extubation

Cardiovascular Management

♦ Hypertension:
  – Depending on how it is defined, hypertension occurs in 30 to
  80% of patients after intracranial surgery. Uncontrolled hypertension increases the risk of intracranial bleeding after craniotomy.
  Neurosurgical patients may have impaired regional or global cerebral autoregulation, such that increases in blood pressure are
  accompanied by significant rises in CBF and ICP. Severe hypertension may displace CBF beyond the autoregulatory plateau,
  where CBF and ICP become pressure-dependent
  – Diagnostic uncertainty may arise because hypertension is a sign
  of increased ICP (Cushing's reflex). An acute intracranial process
  of sufficient magnitude to cause hypertension will typically be
  associated with abnormal clinical findings including decreased
  arousal and pupillary changes, although on occasion hypertension
  precedes any neurologic abnormality. Significant bradycardia or a
  declining heart rate in association with hypertension and new
  unanticipated neurologic findings are highly suggestive of
  intracranial hypertension (*see* Fig. 2)
  – Other potential causes of postoperative hypertension include
  pain, anxiety, shivering, bladder distension, and respiratory depression with hypercapnia and hypoxia. After these possibilities have
  been addressed, it is reasonable to ascribe hypertension to a nonspecific perioperative stress response. Neurologic reassessment
  should be frequent; changes, even subtle, should instantly redirect
  attention to an intracranial process
  – Treatment of hypertension (*see* also Chapter 5) should reduce
  blood pressure without adversely affecting cerebral autoregulatory
  mechanisms, CBF, CMRO2, or ICP:
    • First line agents are β-adrenergic antagonists which can be
    titrated intravenously, such as labetalol, esmolol, and metoprolol.
    • In the presence of refractory hypertension or when heart rate
    prohibits β-blockers, ACE-inhibitor or vasodilators such as

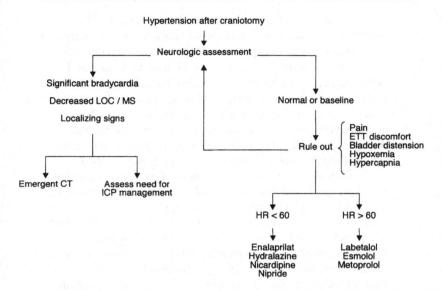

Fig. 2. Management of hypertension in neurosurgical patients.

hydralazine, nicardipine, or nitroprusside are given. The latter
are second line therapies as they dilate cerebral vasculature and
increase ICP. However, the risks of uncontrolled hypertension
and intracranial bleeding in the postoperative setting are
believed to outweigh the possible consequences of drug-
induced cerebral vasodilation. Limited evidence indicates that
enalaprilat, an angiotensin converting enzyme inhibitor, minimally perturbs CBF and ICP. The efficacy of this drug in the
perioperative neurosurgical setting has not been tested
– Hypotension after craniotomy is relatively uncommon (2 to
5%); if severe it may compromise CBF resulting in irreversible
brain injury, especially in the setting of a prior insult. Hypotension
is a correlated with poor outcome after traumatic brain injury.
Hypotension may develop secondary to decreased intravascular
volume (preload), cardiac dysfunction, or inappropriate peripheral
vasodilation (afterload):
    • Common causes of hypovolemia after neurosurgery include
blood loss, osmotic diuresis, insufficient fluid resuscitation, and
diabetes insipidus

- Neurogenic cardiac dysfunction has been described following subarachnoid hemorrhage, intracerebral hemorrhage, traumatic brain injury, and spinal cord injury. Pathophysiology is unclear but may involve massive catecholamine release and adrenergic receptor stimulation, tipping the balance of myocardial oxygen supply and demand. May be clinically latent or manifest as dysrhythmia, hypotension, shock, ST and T-wave abnormalities, troponin release, and global or regional wall motion abnormalities on echocardiography. May coexist with (and is thought to be pathophysiologically linked to) NPE
- Neurogenic shock refers to a pattern of decreased heart rate, blood pressure, and systemic vascular resistance that develops secondary to high thoracic or cervical spinal cord injury Underlying mechanism is sympathetic denervation to the heart and peripheral vasculature. Management includes intravascular fluid resuscitation and enhancing inotropy and peripheral vasoconstriction; dopamine may be a useful first-line agent

– Carotid endarterectomy is associated with significant hemodynamic changes in over 40% of cases
- Hypotensive episodes may reflect ongoing bleeding, myocardial ischemia/infarction, or tension pneumothorax. In some cases, hypotension has been attributed to increased discharge from denuded carotid sinus baroreceptors, resulting in reflex bradycardia and vasodilation
- Hypertension is generally secondary to perioperative catecholamine discharge, however hyperemic cerebral edema may also be a causative factor

– Aggressive hemodynamic support may be needed in the setting of intracranial hypertension or cerebral vasospasm. These therapies usually necessitate placement of intravascular access and monitoring devices (e.g., central venous, pulmonary artery, arterial catheters):
- Commonly used adrenergic agents:
  □ Vasopressors:
    ◊ Phenylephrine, pure α_1 agonist, 10–200 μg/min
    ◊ Norepinephrine, α_1 agonist with some β_1 activity, 0.05–1 μg/kg/min
  □ Inotrope: dobutamine, β_1 and β_2 agonist, 2–20 μg/kg/min
  □ Agents with mixed properties:
    ◊ Dopamine, dose dependent dopamine/β/α agonist, 3–20 μg/kg/min
    ◊ Epinephrine, β and β agonist 0.05–1 μg/kg/min

- Intracranial hypertension. Meeting CPP goals involves a step-wise approach. MAP is usually only marginally increased with intravascular volume loading. However, it is advisable to ensure euvolemia before instituting pharmacologic therapy. Patients with normal left ventricular function are treated with vasopressors initially and inotropic or mixed agents are introduced if further augmentation is needed. Patients with decreased left ventricular function should receive an agent with inotropic properties
- Cerebral vasospasm. Hyperdynamic therapy of cerebral vasospasm couples blood pressure augmentation with intravascular volume expansion. Pharmacologic agents are used as outlined above. Volume expansion should be goal-directed (e.g., specific fluid balance, central venous pressure, or pulmonary artery occlusion pressure endpoints). Adjunctive treatment with the mineralocorticoid analogue fludrocortisone promotes fluid retention

Fluid, Electrolyte, and Endocrine Management

♦ Fluid management after neurosurgery should emphasize adequacy of end-organ perfusion and euvolemia. Perioperative fluid-restrictive strategies aimed at minimizing cerebral edema are ineffective and promote suboptimal oxygen delivery and organ dysfunction. Patients should receive fluids to cover basic metabolic needs, insensible losses, urine output, gastrointestinal output, and any ongoing blood losses:

  − Accurate estimation of intravascular volume in the critically ill may be challenging and should be guided by patterns and trends rather than isolated variables. Commonly used endpoints for fluid resuscitation include:

  − Clinical indicators: Skin perfusion, urine output, heart rate, blood pressure, mentation, fluid balance, weight

  − Physiologic indicators: Central venous pressure, pulmonary artery occlusion pressure, cardiac output

  − Laboratory indicators: Blood urea nitrogen (BUN) to creatinine ratio, urine sodium, echocardiographic data

♦ For uncomplicated brain surgeries, serum osmolality should be maintained in the normal range. Isotonic saline solutions are preferred. Lactated Ringer's, dextrose in water, and hypotonic saline solutions are not appropriate as they may decrease plasma osmolality and promote brain swelling

♦ In patients with cerebral edema related to surgery or trauma, a strategy of increasing serum osmolality reduces brain water content and ICP (*see* Chapter 5). Commonly used agents include mannitol and hypertonic saline solutions. The relative efficacy of these agents for control of ICP has not been clearly established. Mannitol is a diuretic and depletes intravascular volume whereas hypertonic saline solutions are plasma expanders. Repeated administration or infusions or hyperosmolar compounds in the setting of blood–brain barrier dysfunction may lead to solute accumulation in the brain and rebound edema when osmotic therapy is discontinued

♦ Disturbances of water and sodium metabolism (*see* Table 5):
  – Sodium is the principal extracellular cation and accounts for 95% of serum osmolality. In the presence of an intact blood brain barrier, net fluxes of water in and out of the brain are primarily determined by serum sodium concentration
  – Hyponatremia (<135 mmol/L) occurs in up to one third of patients with a neurosurgical disorder. It leads to a net increase in brain water content and can manifest clinically as nausea, seizures, lethargy, or coma. Pseudohyponatremia occurs when hyperproteinemia or hyperlipidemia are severe enough to account for an appreciable part of the volume of plasma in which sodium is dissolved. Hyponatremia may be hyperosmolar or isoosmolar (hyperglycemia, mannitol) but most commonly is hypoosmolar. Hypoosmolar hyponatremia is differentiated on the basis of extracellular fluid volume (*see* Table 6). In the neurosurgical population, common causes of hyponatremia are SIADH and cerebral salt wasting:
    • Management of hyponatremia is directed to the underlying disorder. Correction of chronic hyponatremia should not exceed 12–15 mmol/24 h (risk of osmotic demyelination syndrome). Sodium deficit is determined according to the formula:

$$\text{Na deficit (mmol)} = ([\text{Na}]\ \text{goal (mmol/L)} - [\text{Na}]\ \text{current (mmol/L)}) \times \text{TBW}$$

    Where TBW is total body-water (60% of body weight in the male, 50% in the female)
    • SIADH is characterized by dysregulated hypersecretion of vasopressin. Patients are hyponatremic, euvolemic or midly hypervolemic, and have inappropriately concentrated urine. Commonest causes are malignancies, pulmonary disease, and brain disorders, including tumors, infection, hemorrhages, and

Table 5
Neurosurgical Sodium and Water Abnormalities

	Central diabetes insipidus	*SIADH*	*Cerebral salt wasting*
Typical setting	Pituitary surgery Brain death	Malignancy Meningitis	SAH
Endocrine abnormality	Decreased ADH	Increased ADH	Increased natriuretic peptide
Intravascular volume	Decreased	Normal/increased	Decreased
Urine output	Increased	Normal	Increased
Serum Na (mmol/L)	>145	<135	<135
Serum osmolality	>300	<280	<280
Urine:serum osmolality	<1	>1.5	>1.5
Urine Na (mmol/L)	<10	>20	>40
Management	ADH substitution	Water restriction	Restoration of intravascular volume

SIADH, syndrome of inappropriate antiduiretic hormone secretion; SAH, subarachnoid hemorrhage; ADH, antidiuretic hormone.

trauma; transient SIADH may be observed in the perioperative period. Treatment is fluid restriction. If severe or symptomatic, a loop diuretic and hypertonic saline may be needed. If pathology necessitates high pressure goals (e.g., cerebral vasospasm, cerebral edema, elevated ICP), then hyponatremia is treated with hypertonic saline
• Cerebral salt wasting (CSW) is characterized by abnormal renal sodium excretion in the setting of a brain disorder, most typically subarachnoid hemorrhage. Thought to be mediated by natriuretic peptide release. Patients are hyponatremic, hypovolemic, with inappropriately high urine sodium. CSW is distinguished from SIADH on the basis of decreased intravascular volume. Treatment is correction of fluid and sodium deficit with isotonic or hypertonic saline
• Osmotic demyelination has been observed when chronic hyponatremia is corrected hastily (>20 mml/24 h). Patients

Table 6
Causes of Hyponatremia

Increased ECF	*Normal ECF*	*Decreased ECF*
Congestive heart failure	SIADH	Renal losses
Acute or chronic renal	Drugs	Diuretic excess
failure	Hypothyroidism	Mineralocorticoid deficiency
Nephrotic syndrome	Polydipsia	Salt-losing nephropathy
Cirrhosis	Glucocorticoid	Osmotic diuresis
	deficiency	Extra renal losses
		Cerebral salt wasting
		Vomiting
		Diarrhea
		Third spacing of fluids
		Burns
		Pancreatitis

Abbr: ECF, extracellular fluid; SIADH, syndrome of inappropriate antidiuretic hormone secretion.

present typically with tetraparesis, ophtalmoplegia, ataxia, dysphagia, lethargy, and coma. Lesions have been described in the pons (central pontine myelinolysis), midbrain, subcortical white matter, and are typically irreversible. Treatment is supportive
– Hypernatremia (>145 mmol/L) occurs in 10 to 20% of neurosurgical patients. Clinical manifestations include thirst, ataxia, seizures; and intracranial hemorrhage. Hypernatremic disorders are secondary either to a net loss of water or hypotonic fluid, or to a gain in sodium; management of hypernatremia should consider the underlying mechanism (*see* Table 7)

• Diabetes insipidus (DI) is the most common cause of hypernatremia observed in the neurosurgical setting. It is caused by decreased vasopressin activity. Central (neurogenic) DI occurs with hypothalamic–pituitary dysfunction or injury. Frequent etiologies are tumors, infections, trauma, surgery (hypophysectomy), and brain death. Nephrogenic DI is characterized by diminished renal sensitivity to vasopressin; it is caused by chronic renal disease, electrolyte disturbances, drugs, and certain genetic disorders and not commonly observed in the post-neurosurgical setting:

Table 7
Causes of Hypernatremia

Net water loss	Sodium gain
Diabetes insipidus	Hypertonic saline
Loop diuretics	Primary hyperaldosteronism
Postobstructive diuresis	Cushing's syndrome
Polyuric phase of ATN	Hypertonic dialysis
Vomiting	
Diarrhea	
Enteric fisulas	
Nasogastric drainage	
Burns	
Sweating	

Abbr: ATN, acute tubular necrosis.

- □ Diagnostic criteria for DI include:
  - ◊ Decreased urine osmolality <150 mOsm/kg or specific gravity <1.005)
  - ◊ Increased urine output (>3 mL/kg/h)
  - ◊ Rising serum sodium or hypernatremia (>145 mmol/L)
- • Management goal is to restore normal intravascular volume and serum sodium. Serum sodium, urine osmolality or specific gravity, and urine output should be monitored closely (q 2 to 4 h). Mild presentations may require minimal intervention other than free access to PO fluids. With more severe forms, urine output should be replaced mL for mL with 1/2 normal saline and substitution initiated (starting dose, AVP 5 U subcutaneously q 4 to 6 h). Alternatively, vasopressin may be given as an infusion (dilute AVP 1 U in 1 L 1/2 normal saline, replace urine output mL for mL)
- – Corticosteroids are liberally prescribed in a wide variety of neurosurgical settings. However, evidence-based indications for glucocorticoids in neurosurgery are few (brain tumor-associated edema):
  - • Adverse effects of steroids include hypertension, sodium and water retention, psychosis, stress ulcers, and gastritis, pancreatitis, glucose intolerance, immunosuppression, and hypercoagulability

• Inhibition of endogenous steroid production leads to adrenal insufficiency if corticosteroids are reduced or withdrawn abruptly. Severe adrenal insufficiency may present as lethargy or coma, hypotension, hyponatremia, hyperkalemia, hypoglycemia and fever. Clinical suspicion may be substantiated with random cortisol or ACTH stimulation test. Management is hydrocortisone, 50–100 mg IV q8 h

– Hyperglycemia worsens outcomes after stroke, subarachnoid hemorrhage, and traumatic brain injury. A strategy of aggressive glycemic control has been shown to decrease mortality in critically ill patients. Diabetic and nondiabetic neurosurgical patients frequently present with hyperglycemia because of perioperative catecholamine release, corticosteroids, and infection. Tight insulin regimens should be used to maintain serum glucose in the 80 to 120 mmol/L range

Thromboembolism

♦ Deep venous thrombosis (DVT) occurs in 19 to 50% of patients after neurosurgery. Risk factors are intracranial (vs spinal) surgery, malignant (vs benign) tumors, duration of surgery, the presence of leg weakness, and increased age. Independently of surgery, patients with gliomas have a particularly high risk

♦ Pulmonary embolism (PE) develops in 0.5% of patients undergoing craniotomy and carries a mortality of up to 50%

♦ Clinical findings may be suggestive but are nonspecific. They must be substantiated with Doppler/ultrasound or venography for DVT; V/Q scans, spiral CT scan, or pulmonary angiogram for PE. A negative D-dimer titer rules out thromboembolism in 95% of cases

♦ Prophylaxis with intermittent compression devices decreases risk of DVT by 66% after craniotomy, and the use of enoxaparin combined with elastic stockings was found to be more effective than stockings alone. A recent head-to-head comparison of low-molecular-weight heparin with low-dose unfractionated heparin after intracranial surgery showed equal effectiveness. In prospective controlled trials, risk of intracranial bleeding was not significantly increased by heparin prophylaxis

♦ Management of established DVT or PE after intracranial surgery must be decided on a case-by-case basis. Risk of intracranial bleeding with therapeutic heparin must be weighed against risk of hemodynamic compromise or death from PE. Detailed information on the surgical procedure may aid in estimating the risk of a hemorrhagic complication. Risk/benefit of anticoagulation may swing rapidly in favor of anticoagulation as surgery becomes more remote

Key Points

♦ Goal of neurosurgical intensive care is to prevent, detect, and treat postoperative complications

♦ Initial postoperative management must assess airway, breathing, and hemodynamic function, coupled with a directed neurologic examination

♦ Systemic disturbances such as hypoxemia, hypotension, hyponatremia, hyperglycemia, and hyperthermia adversely affect outcome after cerebral injury and should be aggressively corrected

♦ Delayed awakening after intracranial surgery is a nonspecific response which may signal intracranial hemorrhage, brain edema, anesthetic effects, or a systemic disturbance

♦ Hypertension after intracranial surgery is also nonspecific, associated with intracranial hypertension as well as with pain and perioperative stress responses

♦ Ventilatory weaning and extubation of neurosurgical patients should be preceded by a consideration of level of consciousness, intracranial compliance, bulbar function, and respiratory function

Suggested Reading

Barnett HJM, Taylor DW, Eliasziw M, Fox AJ, Ferguson GG, Haynes RB, et al, for the North American Symptomatic Carotid Endarterectomy Trial Collaborators. Benefit of carotid endarterectomy in patients with symptomatic moderate or severe stenosis. *N Engl J Med* 1998;339:1415–1425.

Brell M, Ibanez J, Caral L, and Ferrer E. Factors influencing surgical complications of intra-axial brain tumours. *Act. Neurochir* (Wien) 2000;142:739–750

Bruder N and Ravussin P. Recovery from anesthesia and postoperative extubation of neurosurgical patients. *J Neurosurg Anesth* 1999;4:282–293.

Geerts WH, Heit JA, Clagett GP, Pineo GF, Colwell CW, Anderson FA Jr, and Wheeler HB. Prevention of venous thromboembolism. *Chest* 2001;119:132S-175S.

Harrigan MR. Cerebral salt wasting syndrome. *Crit Care Clin* 2001; 17:125–138.

Mamminen PH, Raman SK, Boyle K, and El Beheiry H. Early postoperative complications following neurosurgical procedures. *Can J Anaesth* 1999;46:7–14

Molyneux A, Kerr R, Stratton I, Sandercock P, Clarke M, Shrimpton J, and Holman R. International Subarachnoid Aneurysm Trial (ISAT) of neurosurgical clipping versus endovascular coiling in 2143 patients with ruptured intracranial aneurysms: a randomised trial. *Lancet* 2002;360:1267–1274

Namen AM, Ely EW, Tatter SB, Case LD, Lucia MA, Smith A, et al. Predictors of successful extubation in neurosurgical patients. *Am J Respir Crit Care Med* 2001;163:658–664.

North JB, Penhall RK, Hanieh A, Hann CS, Challen RG, and Frewin DB. Postoperative epilepsy: a double-blind trial of phenytoin after craniotomy. *Lancet* 1980;23:384–386.

van den Berghe G, Wouters P, Weekers F, Verwaest C, Bruyninckx F, Schetz M, et al. Intensive insulin therapy in the critically ill patients. *N Engl J Med* 2001;345:1359–1367.

8 Ischemic Stroke

Agnieszka A. Ardelt

Definition of Ischemic Stroke
Transient Ischemic Attack (TIA)

♦ Transient focal neurologic deficit, corresponding to ischemia of an arterial territory in the brain

Ischemic Stroke or Cerebrovascular Accident (CVA)

♦ Focal neurologic deficit, corresponding to an arterial territory infarction (i.e., permanent brain injury):
  – Leading cause of disability
  – Third leading cause of death in the United States
  – Substantial portion of US healthcare expenditure
  – Substantial societal cost because of long-term disability and lost productivity

Mechanisms of Ischemic Stroke
Embolic

♦ Cardiac sources (valves, atria, ventricles, endocardium, aortic arch)
♦ Artery-to-artery embolism
♦ Systemic veins (paradoxical embolism)

Thrombotic (Progressive or Sudden Closure of Vessel Lumen)

♦ Atherosclerosis (large extracranial and intracranial vessels)
♦ Fibromuscular dysplasia
♦ Arteritis

From: *Current Clinical Neurology: Handbook of Neurocritical Care*
Edited by: A. Bhardwaj, M. A. Mirski, and J. A. Ulatowski © Humana Press Inc., Totowa, NJ

> ## Box 1
> ## Pathology of Plaque Rupture
> – Formation of clot on top of plaque
> – Hemorrhage into a plaque and sudden vessel occlusion
> – Progressive thrombosis of the vessel and infarction of the downstream territory
> – Possible embolism of the clot distally and infarction of a smaller area within the vessel's territory
> – Possible watershed, or border zone, infarcts in the setting of systemic hypotension

- Arterial dissection
- Lipohyalinosis (small end arteries)
- Altered blood rheology
- Vasospasm

Hemodynamic

- Relative systemic arterial hypotension in the setting of fixed extracranial or intracranial stenosis

Risk Factors for Ischemic Stroke
Common (Atherosclerotic) Causes of Endothelial Damage (see Box 1)

- Advanced age
- Male sex
- Diabetes mellitus
- Hypertension
- Hypercholesterolemia
- Smoking history
- Coronary artery disease

Rare Causes of Endothelial Damage

- Inflammatory and infectious vasculopathies (e.g., Takayatsu's and giant-cell arteritis, varicella, syphilis)
- Drug-induced vasculopathies (e.g., cocaine, amphetamines)
- Rare, inherited conditions such as fibromuscular dysplasia and Fabry's Disease
- Dissection of carotid or vertebral arteries, either purely traumatic or associated with predisposing conditions such as collagen vascular disorders

Lacunar Disease

♦ Related to long-standing hypertension
♦ Lipohyalinosis of penetrating arteries
♦ Thrombosis of penetrating arteries
♦ Involves deep-brain regions, such as the basal ganglia and the pons
♦ Stereotyped clinical syndromes, referred to as lacunar syndromes

Cardiac Sources

♦ Atherosclerotic disease of the aortic arch
♦ Atrial fibrillation and other dysrhythmias
♦ Valvular heart disease
♦ Low ejection fraction with wall motion abnormalities
♦ Acute myocardial infarction
♦ Patent foramen ovale in association with atrial septal aneurysm
♦ Atrial septal defects and patent foramen ovale in the setting of systemic vein thrombosis (paradoxical embolism)

Hypercoagulable States (Also Likely to Lead to Venous Infarcts)

♦ Anti-phospholipid antibody syndrome
♦ Pregnancy/oral contraceptives
♦ Systemic cancer
♦ Crohn's disease
♦ Genetic deficiencies (e.g., Leiden factor V, prothrombin 20210, protein C, protein S, anti-thrombin III)

Conditions Affecting Blood Rheology

♦ Sickle cell anemia
♦ Increased viscosity (e.g., Waldenstrom's, multiple myeloma)
♦ Polycythemia
♦ Thrombocytosis
♦ Spherocytosis
♦ High leukocrit (e.g., leukemia)

The Patient With Acute Neurologic Deficit:
Basic Concepts
Differential Diagnosis

♦ Ischemic stroke
♦ Ischemic stroke mimics:
  – Masses:
    • Abscess
    • Subdural and epidural hematomas/subarachnoid hemorrhage

- Tumors
- Giant aneurysms
- Arteriovenous malformations (AVMs) and other vascular malformations
  - Intracerebral hemorrhage
  - Encephalitis/cerebritis
  - Seizure/Todd's paralysis
  - Migraine
  - Metabolic (hypo- or hyperglycemia)
  - Deficit from a previous stroke or injury made worse by general medical condition such as infection or iatrogenic reasons such as general anesthesia
♦ Cerebral venous/sinus thrombosis

Clinical Stroke Syndromes

Arterial supply is relatively stereotyped, and ischemia in specific territories supplied by particular arteries leads to recognizable clinical syndromes (*see* Fig. 1)
♦ Hemispheric lesion (internal carotid artery plus anterior cerebral and middle cerebral arteries):
  - Dominant: Aphasia, contralateral motor weakness, contralateral sensory loss, contralateral visual field cut, poor conjugate gaze to the contralateral side, troubles with calculations, reading, writing
  - Nondominant: difficulty with visuo-spatial construction, contralateral motor and sensory deficit, neglect syndromes, somatosensory and visual extinction, mental status changes, contralateral visual field cut, poor conjugate gaze to the contralateral side
♦ Posterior cerebral artery:
  - Dominant: Contralateral field cut (may be macular-sparing), alexia without agraphia, achromatopsia, decreased visual recognition of objects, contralateral sensory loss
  - Nondominant: contralateral visual field cut, contralateral visual neglect, contralateral sensory loss
♦ Vertebrobasilar system:
  - Vertigo, nausea, vomiting, diplopia, ataxia, gait difficulty, weakness and numbness (may involve all limbs), crossed motor and sensory findings, loss of consciousness, bilateral visual field deficits, blindness
♦ Lacunar syndromes (*see* Box 2)

> ### Box 2
> ### Lacunar Syndromes
>
> ♦ Pure contralateral hemisensory loss (face-arm-leg):
>   – Thalamus
> ♦ Pure contralateral motor weakness (face-arm-leg):
>   – Internal capsule
>   – Pons
> ♦ Ataxic hemiparesis:
>   – Contralateral internal capsule
>   – Contralateral pons
> ♦ Dysarthria-clumsy hand:
>   – Contralateral internal capsule
>   – Contralateral pons

Imaging

♦ Head computed tomography (CT):
  – Rules out hemorrhage acutely
  – Can show early signs of stroke, within hours of onset (blurring of gray-white, sulcal effacement)
  – Can show dense vessel sign (calcified clot in a vessel)
  – Can show atherosclerosis (calcified blood vessel walls)
  – Rules out most tumors, abscess (with contrast)
  – Visualizes sinuses and mastoids (as a source of abscess, cerebritis)
♦ Magnetic resonance imaging (MRI):
  – Shows hemorrhage (gradient echo)
  – Shows acute infarct as early as minutes after onset (bright signal on diffusion and black signal on apparent diffusion coefficient [ADC] sequences)
  – Can delineate the ischemic penumbra (i.e., the territory at risk for further infarction)
  – Can show chronic edema, ischemia (fluid attenuated inversion recovery [FLAIR], T2 sequences)
  – Can identify masses (e.g., tumors, abscess [T1 with gadolinium])
♦ Magnetic resonance angiography (MRA)
  – Evaluates intracranial vasculature/circle of Willis
  – Evaluates extracranial vasculature (neck MRA with gadolinium)
  – Delineates aneurysms

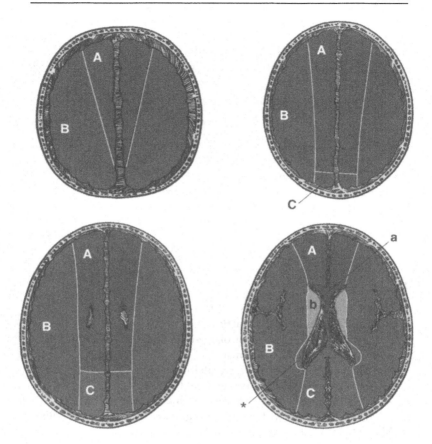

Fig. 1. Vascular territories in the brain (reproduced from Osborn, 1994, with permission). A = Anterior cerebral artery; a = medial lenticulo-striate and callosal perforating arteries from anterior cerebral artery; B = middle cerebral artery; b = lateral lenticulostriate branches from middle cerebral artery; C = posterior cerebral artery; c = thalamic and midbrain perforating arteries from posterior cerebral artery; D = superior cerebellar arteries; E = basilar artery perforating branches; F = posterior inferior cerebellar artery; G = anterior inferior cerebellar artery; * = anterior choroidal and anterior thalamoperforating arteries.

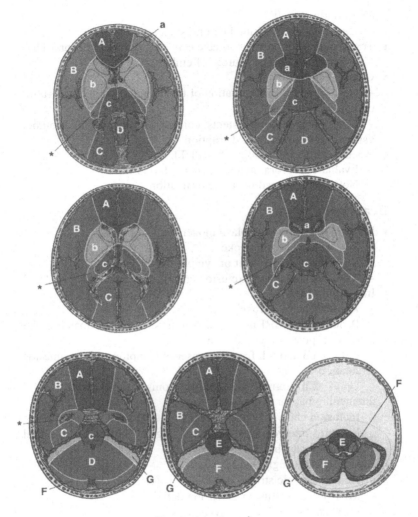

Fig. 1. *(continued)*

♦ Transcranial doppler (TCD):
  – Determines velocity through intracranial vessels as a marker of vessel stenosis/occlusion
  – Determination of collateral circulation in vessel occlusion
  – Detects emboli
  – Determines of physiologic importance of a patent foramen ovale (with bubble study)

♦ Carotid ultrasound:
  – Determines extracranial carotid stenosis, occlusion
♦ Transesophageal or transthoracic echocardiogram (TEE or TTE):
  – Determines cardiac sources of embolism
♦ Cerebral angiogram:
  – Gold standard for evaluation of the cerebral vasculature, ruling out aneurysms
  – Used when deploying stents, coils or for intraarterial thrombolysis and mechanical clot disruption
♦ Positron emission tomography (PET):
  – Evaluates cerebral metabolism and blood flow
  – Not routinely used in stroke evaluation

Treatment Options

♦ Intravenous (IV) tissue plasminogen activator (tPA):
  – For acute ischemic stroke
  – Within 3 h of the onset of symptoms
  – Rigid inclusion and exclusion criteria (*see* Box 4)
♦ Intra-arterial (IA) tPA:
  – Acute ischemic stroke
  – Patients with MRI-proven diffusion-perfusion mismatch in the anterior or posterior circulation
  – Between 3 and 6 h from the onset of symptoms in the anterior circulation
  – Up to 48 h from the onset of symptoms in cases of life-threatening basilar occlusion
  – Inclusion and exclusion criteria similar to those for IV tPA
  – Requires interventional neuroradiological staffing and cerebral angiography capability
♦ Blood pressure augmentation:
  – Acute ischemic stroke
  – MRI-proven diffusion-perfusion deficit
  – Intravenous fluids or neosynephrine
  – Goal is a 10–20% augmentation of blood pressure over patient's baseline, the desired blood pressure range to be individualized, for 24 h, or longer if deficit improves; such patients may be transitioned to postoperative midodrine if they continue to require blood pressure augmentation
  – Ischemic cardiac disease is a relative contraindication

- Aortic dissection, acute myocardial infraction, hypertensive encephalopathy, congestive heart failure and acute renal dysfunction secondary to hypertension are contraindications
♦ Heparin:
  - Studies have failed to establish any benefit of fractionated or unfractionated heparin in acute stroke
  - Increased risk of bleeding with IV heparin in acute stroke
  - May be appropriate in selected patients:
    • Ongoing posterior circulation ischemia, such as basilar thrombosis, in patients who are not candidates for other interventions
    • Small stroke or transient ischemic attack in the setting of atrial fibrillation or acute myocardial infarction
    • Crescendo TIAs
  - The decision to heparinize (and when to heparinize) post-stroke in the above settings is individualized. Patients with smaller infarctions, less than one third the middle cerebral artery territory, for example, may be less likely to sustain a hemorrhagic conversion of the ischemic stroke. Patients with amyloid angiopathy, on the other hand, may be more likely to bleed while anticoagulated. Patients with infectious endocarditis and embolic strokes are also at higher risk of intracerebral hemorrhage. Acute heparinization may be a bridge to chronic therapy with coumadin
♦ Warfarin (coumadin):
  - Chronic atrial fibrillation
  - As a bridge to carotid endarterectomy
  - Stroke in the setting of low-ejection fraction
  - Carotid and vertebral dissection
  - Hypercoagulability syndromes
♦ Anti-platelet agents:
  - Mainstay of acute and chronic treatment of stroke and TIA
  - Include aspirin, aspirin/dipyridamole, clopidogrel, and ticlodipine (less used currently secondary to side effects)
  - Ongoing controversies:
    • Optimal dose of aspirin
    • Whether dual agent (combination) therapy offers additional benefit
♦ Surgical and interventional therapy:
  - Carotid endarterectomy:

- Gold standard for treatment of symptomatic extracranial carotid stenosis
- Appropriate in some settings for treatment of severe asymptomatic extracranial carotid stenosis
  - Stenting and angioplasty:
    - May be used in specific cases to open stenotic intracranial vessels responsible for ischemic symptoms
    - In select patients may be used to open stenotic extracranial vessels (e.g., radiation carotid vasculopathy)
  - Surgical arterial bypass:
    - Used in select cases to provide perfusion to an area threatened by a stenosis that is otherwise inaccessible (e.g., external carotid to internal carotid anastomosis)
  - Hemicraniectomy:
    - Reserved for patients with projected relatively good functional outcome who are experiencing life-threatening edema with impending herniation in the days immediately post-stroke
    - May not improve functional outcome *per se* but may save the patient's life

The Patient With Acute Focal Neurologic Deficit: *General Protocols*

♦ Rule out stroke mimics
♦ Determine if the patient meets criteria for acute therapy
♦ Determine if the patient needs to be admitted to the intensive care unit (ICU) (*see* Box 3)

The Patient With Acute Focal Neurologic Deficit: *Specific Protocol*

The Patient with Acute Focal Deficit Presenting Within 3 h of Onset (Possible Candidate for IV tPA)

♦ History:
  - Determine the time of onset
  - Determine if the patient had a seizure or suffers from a seizure disorder
  - Determine if patient meets inclusion and exclusion criteria for IV tPA (*see* Box 4)
♦ Physical exam and laboratory work:
  - Obtain immediate blood glucose
  - Obtain blood pressure measurement. Control systolic blood pressure >180 mmHg

> **Box 3**
> **Criteria for Admission of Stroke Patients to the ICU**
> ♦ Post IV or IA tPA
> ♦ Patients with large hemispheric stroke, in whom impending mental status decline and loss of protective airway reflexes is of a concern
> ♦ Patients with basilar thrombosis or top of the basilar syndrome
> ♦ Patients with crescendo TIAs
> ♦ Patients requiring blood pressure augmentation for a documented area of hypoperfusion
> ♦ Patients requiring IV blood pressure or heart rate control
> ♦ Patients requiring q 1–2 h neurological evaluation depending on symptom fluctuation or if ongoing ischemia is suspected
> ♦ Patients with worsening neurological status

  – Determine the NIH–Stroke Scale (NIH–SS) (*see* Box 5)
  – Send STAT laboratories including heme-8, activated partial thromboplastin time ratio (aPTTr), inernational normalized ratio (INR), chemistry panel, arterial blood gas (ABG)
♦ Procedures and studies:
  – Insert 2 peripheral IVs, at least 20 gage
  – Insert Foley catheter
  – Head CT STAT
  – Electrocardiogram (EKG)
♦ Re-establish tPA eligibility when all the data is collected
♦ Obtain consent for IV tPA (major benefit: recanalization of blood vessel and improved functional outcome; major risk: bleeding systemically and intracranially, which can be fatal)
♦ Administer IV tPA (*see* Box 6)

The Patient With Acute Focal Deficit Presenting Between 3 and 6 h After Onset

♦ Patients presenting between 3 and 6 h post onset of symptoms may qualify for IA administration of tPA, if neurointerventional services are available. A STAT MRI of the brain with diffusion and perfusion sequences needs to be obtained to determine if there is an area of mismatch (i.e., a territory at risk for infarction). After the MRI, eligibility for IA tPA needs to be determined using the IV tPA criteria as the basis, in discussion with the neurointerventional radiologist who will be performing the procedure

Box 4
Intravenous tPA Inclusion and Exclusion Criteria

♦ Inclusion criteria:
  – Age > 18 yr
  – Clinical diagnosis of ischemic stroke causing measurable neurologic deficit (usually NIH-SS 4–22)
  – Well-established onset of stroke, within 180 min of treatment
♦ Exclusion criteria:
  – Strong Contraindications
   • Rapidly improving symptoms
   • Stroke or head trauma within past 3 mo
   • Major surgery within last 14 d
   • History of intracranial hemorrhage
   • Sustained systolic blood pressure >185 mmHg
   • Sustained diastolic blood pressure >110 mmHg
   • Aggressive treatment necessary to lower blood pressure
   • Symptoms suggest subarachnoid hemorrhage
   • Gastrointestinal or urinary tract hemorrhage within 21 d
   • Arterial puncture at noncompressible site within 7 d
   • Received heparin within 48 h and had elevated PTT
   • Platelet count <100,000
  – Relative contraindications:
   • Seizure at stroke onset (postictal presentation may mimic stroke syndrome)
   • Serum glucose <50 mg/dL or >400 mg/dL
   • Hemorrhagic eye disorder
   • Myocardial infarction in the prior 6 wk
   • Suspected septic embolism
   • Infective endocarditis
   • INR >1.7

The Patient With Acute Focal Deficit not Eligible for IV or IA tPA, Hypertensive Therapy, and ICU Admission

♦ Admit to the hospital, preferably to a "stroke unit", where a multidisciplinary staff is specialized in the care of patients with neurologic disease (*see* Box 8 for admission orders)
♦ Unless contraindicated, aspirin 325 mg, should be administered
♦ Hypertension should not be aggressively treated, unless BP is sustained above 220/120 mmHg

Box 5
NIH–Stroke Scale

♦ 1A. Level of consciousness:
- 0: Alert
- 1: Drowsy
- 2: Stuporous
- 3: Comatose

♦ 1B. Level of consciousness questions:
- 0: Answers both correctly
- 1: Answers one correctly
- 2: Answers both incorrectly

♦ 1C. Level of consciousness commands:
- 0: Obeys both commands correctly
- 1: Obeys one correctly
- 2: Does neither correctly

♦ 2. Best gaze:
- 0: Normal
- 1: Partial gaze palsy
- 2: Forced deviation

♦ 3. Visual fields:
- 0: No visual loss
- 1: Partial hemianopsia
- 2: Complete hemianopsia
- 3: Bilateral hemianopsia

♦ 4. Facial paresis:
- 0: Normal movement
- 1: Minor paresis
- 2: Partial paresis
- 3: Complete palsy

♦ 5–8. Right/left arm/leg motor:
- 0: No drift

- 1: Drift
- 2: Some effort against gravity
- 3: No effort against gravity
- 4: No movement
- x: Untestable

♦ 9. Limb ataxia:
- 0: Absent
- 1: Present in one limb
- 2: Present in two or more limbs
- x: Untestable

♦ 10. Sensory:
- 0: Normal
- 1: Partial loss
- 2: Dense loss

♦ 11. Best language:
- 0: No aphasia
- 1: Mild to moderate aphasia
- 2: Severe aphasia
- 3: Mute

♦ 12. Dysarthria:
- 0: Normal articulation
- 1: Mild to moderate dysarthria
- 2: Unintelligible
- x: Untestable

♦ 13. Neglect/inattention:
- 0: No neglect
- 1: Partial neglect
- 2: Complete neglect

Total Score (0–42)

> ## Box 6
> ## IV tPA Administration
>
> ♦ If a patient meets the criteria for IV tPA, the appropriate dose is infused. Ten percent of the dose is given as a bolus over 1 min, and the rest is infused over one hour, for a total dose of 0.9 mg/kg, maximum 90 kg. Because of the increased chance of bleeding with tPA, patients that have been treated are subject to specific post-tPA orders (*see* Box 7). Such patients should be observed in a high-acuity setting such as an ICU for at least 24 h

♦ Neurological examination should be repeated every 4 h and any acute changes emergently investigated
♦ Immediate evaluation of pulmonary aspiration risk. NPO consideration and possible endotracheal intubation if imminent aspiration risk
♦ Special attention should be paid to providing deep venous thrombosis (DVT) prophylaxis, gastrointestinal (GI) ulcer prophylaxis, and a stool softener
♦ Meticulous skin care and frequent turning of the patient should be used to decrease the incidence of pressure ulcers
♦ Blood sugars have to be judiciously controlled, and elevations in body temperature aggressively treated as both hyperglycemia and hyperthermia worsen outcome in brain injury
♦ Speech/language, physical, and occupational therapists and social workers should be involved in the care of the stroke patient as soon as possible after admission
♦ Stroke patients should be thoroughly investigated to determine the etiology of the ischemia/infarct in order to offer appropriate acute and preventative therapy

Differential Diagnosis and Approach to the Stroke Patient With a Deteriorating Neurological Exam

Cerebral Edema

♦ Usually peaks between 48 and 72 h after stroke
♦ Diagnosed with a head CT without contrast
♦ Admit to the ICU
♦ Endotracheal intubation if necessary
♦ Correct metabolic abnormalities, specifically ensure normonatremia (Na^+ 135–145)
♦ Use mannitol as required for herniation

Box 7
Post IV tPA Orders

♦ Admit to a monitored setting
♦ Bleeding precautions
♦ Monitor blood pressure and neurological checks q1h × 24h
♦ No aspirin or heparin for 24 h.
♦ No invasive procedures for 24 h including Foley catheter, NG tube, arterial sticks or IM injections
♦ IV fluids: Normal saline (1.0–1.5 mL/Kg/h)
♦ Bed rest for 24 h.
♦ Obtain head CT STAT if neurological exam worsens to rule out intracranial hemorrhage. If intracranial hemorrhage is present, stop tPA infusion, administer fresh frozen plasma and cryoprecipitate, and obtain neurosurgical consultation

♦ If edema is life-threatening, and patient has otherwise potential for a good functional recovery, consider decompressive hemicraniectomy
♦ Steroids are not effective for cytotoxic edema, and may make brain injury greater by worsening blood sugar control

Hemorrhagic Conversion

♦ More likely to occur with large hemispheric strokes
♦ Diagnosed with head CT
♦ Care as outlined above for edema

New or Progressing Ischemic Stroke

♦ If early, may not be seen on head CT and may require an MRI
♦ Treatment for acute stroke as outlined throughout this chapter

Seizure/Postictal

♦ Patients with ischemic stroke are not usually treated with empiric anti-epileptic medications
♦ If seizure is suspected, a head CT should be done STAT to rule out edema and hemorrhage, and metabolic abnormalities should be ruled out, especially hypo- or hyperglycemia
♦ If seizure is strongly suspected, an EEG should be done, or if an EEG is not immediately available the patient should be loaded with antiepileptic medications, usually either dilantin or valproic acid, IV load 15–20 mg/kg

Box 8
Ward Admission Orders for Patients
With Stroke and TIA

♦ Admit to monitored setting
♦ Cardiac monitor, pulse oximetry
♦ Peripheral IV access
♦ IV Fluids: NS +/– KCl (20–40 mEq/L)
♦ Chest x-ray, EKG
♦ NPO except medications
♦ Bed rest, side rails up
♦ Foley catheter, strict I/Os
♦ Vital signs q 4 h
♦ Neurological checks q 4 h
♦ Stockings and sequential compression devices to lower limbs
♦ Accu-checks/strict sliding scale insulin (e.g., starting at 110)
♦ Medications:
  – Colace 100 mg PO bid
  – Zantac 150 mg PO bid
  – Aspirin 325 PO qd or other appropriate agent
  – Heparin 5000 U SQ bid
  – Tylenol 650 mg q 4–6 PRN for pain or temperature >38.0
♦ Order:
  – Labs: Heme-8, complete metabolic panel, PT, PTT, urinalysis
  – Tests: TEE (or TTE), MRI/A, carotid U/S
  – Physical and occupational therapy and rehabilitation consults
  – Speech and swallowing evaluation

Metabolic Derangement

♦ STAT accu-check to rule out hypoglycemia
♦ Appropriate laboratory work-up to rule out hypo or hyper-natremia, -calcemia; hypercarbia or hypoxia; rising blood urea nitrogen (BUN) and creatinine; thyroid or liver dysfunction
♦ Serum drug level analysis

Infection

♦ Appropriate work up includes cultures (i.e., blood, sputum, urine), urinalysis, chest x-ray; a lumbar puncture (LP) is done if clinically indicated

♦ Attention should be paid to indwelling devices (central lines, urinary catheters) and such devices should be removed or changed if clinically indicated

♦ In patients with nasogastric tubes, sinusitis should be considered as a source of infection

Etiological Work up of Patients With Stroke/TIA

Laboratory Workup

♦ Fasting cholesterol, homocysteine (correlates with increased stroke risk and may be treated easily with folate), rapid plasma reagin (RPR) to rule out syphilis and related vasculopathy; collagen vascular disease and hypercoagulable disorders screening in selected patients (e.g., those under 45 yr of age)

Imaging Studies

♦ EKG, telemetry, and TEE to rule out cardiac and aortic arch sources of embolism

♦ Brain MRI with diffusion and MRA

♦ Carotid ultrasound to rule out extracranial carotid disease

♦ Neck MRA, aortic arch and cerebral angiogram, TCD as clinically indicated

Stroke Care After the Acute Event

♦ Select stroke patients may need to undergo placement of a tracheostomy or a percutaneous esophagogastrostomy tube. In some patients, these devices may be temporary and may eventually be removed as swallowing function and protective airway reflexes return

♦ All stroke patients should receive aggressive occupational and physical therapy, and modification of risk factors should be undertaken as soon as possible (e.g., blood pressure control, blood sugar control, stopping smoking, initiating diet, exercise and lipid-lowering therapy). Some patients may require long-term intensive inpatient rehabilitation

♦ Treatment with anti-platelet agents or coumadin is continued, and other treatment options such as stents or angioplasty should be considered in select patients. All patients are scheduled for post-hospitalization outpatient follow-up

♦ Finally, select patients and their families may benefit from social and psychological support, and patients are provided with a list of such resources in the geographical area

Key Points

♦ Acute onset of focal neurologic deficit has a differential diagnosis, with ischemic stroke and intracerebral hemorrhage highest on the differential. A noncontrast heat CT effectively rules out hemorrhage

♦ Patients presenting with an acute onset of focal neurologic deficit should be speedily evaluated, and if their deficit is most likely ischemic in nature, all efforts are made to administer IV tPA. If patients are not candidates for IV tPA, other acute treatment modalities such as IA tPA, stenting, angioplasty, or blood pressure augmentation are considered

♦ All patients with TIA or stroke should be investigated thoroughly to determine the etiology of the TIA or stroke. Risk factors for stroke are determined and modifiable risk factors are treated

♦ All efforts should be made to keep the stroke patient normonatremic, normoglycemic, and euthermic. Patients should receive DVT and GI prophylaxis, and decubitous ulcers should be prevented. Possible infections are investigated and treated. Physical and occupational therapy should be started as soon as the patient is medically stable

♦ Neurological worsening in stroke patients is thoroughly investigated, and there is a low threshold for admission to an ICU setting

Suggested Reading

Caplan, LR. *Stroke: A Clinical Approach.* Butterworth-Heinemann, Woburn, MA: 2000.

Osborn, AG. *Diagnostic Neuroradiology,* Mosby, St. Louis, MO: 1994.

9 Cerebral Venous Sinus Thrombosis

Connie L. Chen

Epidemiology

- Incidence:
  - Incidence unknown
  - Women > men
  - Mean age < 40 yr in multiple study series
- Population at risk:
  - Women during puerperium or oral contraceptive (OCP) use
  - Patients with underlying risk factors (*see* "Risk Factors")
- Risk factors:
  - Dehydration
  - Pregnancy
  - Infection
  - Blood dyscrasias (including sickle cell)
  - Cardiac disease
  - Diabetes
  - Behçet's disease
  - Collagen vascular disease
  - Inflammatory bowel disease
  - Malignancy
  - Hereditary prothrombotic conditions
  - Nephrotic syndrome
  - Paroxysmal nocturnal hemoglobinuria
  - Head trauma
- Poor prognosticators:
  - Infancy or advanced age
  - Initial presentation of coma, focal neurologic signs
  - High intracranial pressure (ICP)
  - Hemorrhagic infarcts

From: *Current Clinical Neurology: Handbook of Neurocritical Care*
Edited by: A. Bhardwaj, M. A. Mirski, and J. A. Ulatowski © Humana Press Inc., Totowa, NJ

- Thrombosis of deep venous system
- Development of pulmonary embolisms
♦ Clot location:
  - Sagittal (70–85%) and lateral sinuses (70%)
  - Deep venous system less frequent
♦ Pathophysiology:
  - Venous clot leads to venous outflow obstruction, white matter edema, and venous infarct
♦ Mortality:
  - 5.5–18%

Clinical Presentation

♦ Onset:
  - Acute to subacute
♦ Symptoms:
  - Variable, may include[a]:
    • Headache (95%)
    • Seizures (47%)
    • Focal deficit (46%)
    • Paresis (43%)
    • Papilledema (41%)
    • Impaired consciousness (39%)
    • Isolated increased intracranial pressure (20%)
    • Impaired vision/hemianopsia (16%)
    • Coma (15%)
    • Transient ischemic attack (14%)
    • Brainstem/cerebellar signs(12%)
  [a]de Bruijn et al, Cerebral Venous Sinus Thrombosis Study Group
♦ Laboratories:
  - CSF profile may include:
    • Normal (15%)
    • Elevated pressure
    • High protein
    • Pleocytosis
    • High red blood cell count
♦ Radiology:
  - Head computed tomography (CT) without contrast:
    • Cord sign (hyperdensity of thrombosed sinuses and veins; 20–55%)
    • Edema
    • Venous infarct
    • Intracranial hemorrhage (ICH)

- Head CT with contrast:
  - "Empty delta" sign (20%)
  - Normal (20%)
  - Edema
  - Venous infarct
  - ICH
- Magnetic resonance imaging (MRI)/magnetic resonance venogram (MRV):
  - Edema
  - Infarct of posterior temporal lobe, thalamus, periventricular white matter, corpus striatum, superior cerebellum
  - ICH
  - Gadolinium enhancement of venous infarct
  - Unilateral or bilateral parenchymal involvement near midline
  - Venous sinus flow void
- Cerebral angiogram, gold standard
◆ Adverse associated events:
  - Herniation
  - Pulmonary embolism
  - Dural AV fistulas
  - Death

Differential Diagnosis

◆ Diagnosis:
  - Demonstration of thrombus via neuroimaging
  - Search must be undertaken for underlying risk factors
◆ Differential:
  - Arterial stroke
  - Hemorrhagic infarct from other etiology
  - Neoplasm

Management

◆ History and physical examination:
  - Inclusion of cerebral venous sinus thrombosis (CVST)
    - Presence of underlying risk factors
    - Any one of signs/symptoms present
  - Suggests exclusion of CVST:
    - Absence of any signs or symptoms
◆ Studies:
  - Radiology:
    - MRI/MRV or head CT with/out contrast (if MRI/V not available)

- Cerebral angiogram, if high clinical suspicion and above studies negative
- Absence of sinus thrombosis after all neuroimaging suggests exclusion of CVST
- Procedures (if thrombus found):
  - Lumbar puncture if suspicion of infectious component
- Laboratory Investigations (if thrombus found):
  - Evaluate for underlying risk factors:
    - Factor V Leiden
    - Antithrombin III, Protein S and C
    - Activated protein C resistance
    - Anticardiolipin antibodies
    - β-hCG if female

Treatment

- Monitoring:
  - Neurologic exam for signs of elevated ICP (somnolence, Cushing's response, cranial nerve palsies)
  - ICP monitoring (SA bolt, intraventricular catheter or cerebral tissue monitor) if there is concern for herniation
- Supportive:
  - Consider ICU monitoring
  - Aspiration precautions
  - Aggressive IV hydration
  - Withdrawal of OCPs
- Pharmacologic:
  - Limited clinical studies
  - Heparin remains controversial, but is standard of care:
    - Intravenous unfractionated heparin followed by warfarin for 3–6 mo:
      - Goal APTT 80–100 s
      - Intravenous heparin use has been shown to be safe even in ICH patients
      - Low-molecular-weight heparin followed by warfarin was not found to have improvement on outcome
  - Second line therapy:
    - Direct thrombolytic therapy:
      - Limited studies
      - No shown improvement in morbidity or mortality
      - Increased bleeding risk

Key Points

♦ CVST presents with many different symptoms, nonfocal to focal neurologic signs
♦ High-risk patients include women in peurperium, or with OCP use, and a multitude of underlying medical conditions
♦ Diagnosis is made radiographically
♦ Once diagnosed, underlying risk factors are investigated
♦ Treatment for CVST remains unfractionated heparin, even when patients have ICH

Suggested Reading

Allroggen H and Abbott RJ. Cerebral venous sinus thrombosis. *Postgrad Med J* 2000;76:12–15.

Bousser M. Cerebral venous thrombosis. *Stroke* 1999;30:481–483.

Connor SEJ and Jarosz JM. Magnetic resonance imaging of cerebral venous sinus thrombosis. *Clin Radiol* 2002;57:449–461.

de Bruijn SFTM and de Haan RJ, Stam J for the Cerebral Venous Sinus Thrombosis Study Group. Clinical features and prognostic factors of cerebral venous sinus thrombosis in a prospective series of 59 patients. *J Neurol Neurosurg Psych* 2001;70:105–108.

de Bruijn SFTM and Stam J for the Cerebral Venous Sinus Thrombosis Study Group. Randomized, placebo-controlled trial of anticoagulant treatment with low-molecular-weight heparin for cerebral sinus thrombosis. *Stroke* 1999;30:484–488.

Einhäupl KM, Villringer A, Schmiedek P, et al. Heparin treatment in sinus venous thrombosis. *Lancet* 1991;338:597–600.

Fink JN and McAuley DL. Cerebral venous sinus thrombosis: a diagnostic challenge. *Int Med J* 2001;31:384–390.

Frey JL, Muro JG, Jahnke HK, et al. Cerebral venous thrombosis-combined intrathrombus rtPA and intravenous heparin. *Stroke* 1999;3 0489–494.

Kimber J. Cerebral venous sinus thrombosis. *Quart J Med* 2002; 95:137–142.

10 Brain Tumors

Agnieszka A. Ardelt

Clinical Presentation

♦ Clinical presentation depends on the location of the tumor within the brain.

Symptoms and Signs

Headache

♦ As a result of increased intracranial pressure (ICP) from mass effect or hydrocephalus; local irritation or invasion of structures containing pain fibers (e.g., dura, periosteum, blood vessels)
♦ May have tension or migraine characteristics
♦ May occur when coughing or bending over, suggesting elevated ICP
♦ May be associated with nausea and vomiting, suggesting elevated ICP
♦ Classically worse upon awakening because of enhanced edema in prolonged supine position

Progressive Focal Neurologic Deficit

♦ Relates to the location of tumor and the neurologic function subserved by that territory
♦ May progress acutely if there is hemorrhage into the tumor or if edema surrounding the tumor reaches a critical mass; presentation may suggest acute stroke

From: *Current Clinical Neurology: Handbook of Neurocritical Care*
Edited by: A. Bhardwaj, M. A. Mirski, and J. A. Ulatowski © Humana Press Inc., Totowa, NJ

Mental Status Changes

♦ Hydrocephalus
♦ Mass effect on the contralateral hemisphere
♦ Direct involvement of the brain stem reticular activating system

Papilledema

♦ Secondary to increased ICP (long-standing)

Seizures

♦ If tumor is supratentorial involving the cerebral cortex or irritating the cortex from mass effect or edema

World Health Organization (WHO) Classification of Brain Tumors

♦ Classification is based on histopathology
♦ Grading is used for prognosis: the higher the grade the poorer the prognosis

Neuroepithelial Tissue Tumors

♦ Astrocytic tumors (derived from brain astrocytes):
  – Diffuse astrocytoma (WHO grade II):
    • Young adults, 30–40 yr old, mean age 34 yr
    • Most located supratentorially
    • Usually no gadolinium enhancement on magnetic resonance imaging (MRI)
    • Survival 6–8 yr after surgical resection
    • Younger age and gross total tumor resection result in a more favorable prognosis
  – Anaplastic astrocytoma (WHO grade III):
    • Mean age 41 yr old
    • Male predominance (M:F ratio 1.8:1)
    • Similar locations to diffuse astrocytomas
    • Gadolinium-enhancing on MRI, but usually not ring-enhancing
    • Survival 2–5 yr after surgery
    • Progression to glioblastoma portends a poor prognosis
    • Presence of an oligodendroglial component improves prognosis with survival >7 yr after surgery
    • Younger age, high functional status preoperatively, and gross total resection yield a better prognosis

- Glioblastoma (WHO grade IV):
  - 12–15% of all intracranial tumors
  - 50–60% of all astrocytic tumors
  - Age range 45–70 yr old, mean 53 yr
  - Most frequent location in hemispheric subcortical white matter
  - Usually ring-enhancing on MRI with gadolinium
  - "Butterfly glioma": tumor extension through the corpus callosum
  - Arise either as primary tumors (older patients) or on transformation of anaplastic astrocytoma (younger patients)
  - Survival <1 yr
  - Younger age and total resection have a more favorable prognosis
- Pilocytic astrocytoma :
  - Predominantly pediatric tumor, more well-circumscribed than the diffusely infiltrating astrocytomas
- Pleomorphic xanthoastrocytoma :
  - Rare neoplasm, usually slow-growing but may undergo malignant progression
- Desmoplastic cerebral astrocytoma of infancy
- Subependymal giant cell astrocytoma:
  - Benign, develops in patients with tuberous sclerosis
- Oligodendroglial tumors:
  - Oligodendroglioma (WHO grade II):
    - Slow growing, frequently calcified
    - Peak incidence 4th–6th decade, mean 42.6 yr
    - 50–65% located in frontal lobes
    - Most commonly presents with seizures and headaches
    - May have hyperintensity (calcium) on computerized tomography (CT) and may have a heterogeneous signal (hemorrhage, cystic degeneration) on MRI
    - Median survival 3–5 yr after surgery
    - More favorable prognosis with younger age, high functional score, postoperative irradiation, and lack of contrast enhancement
  - Anaplastic oligoastrocytoma (WHO grade III):
    - Mean age 48.7 yr
    - Prognosis less favorable than oligodendroglioma
- Mixed gliomas:
  - Oligoastrocytoma (WHO grade II)
  - Anaplastic oligoastrocytoma (WHO grade III):

- ◆ Ependymal tumors:
  - − Ependymoma (WHO grade II):
    - • May develop in children and adults
    - • 6–12% of all intracranial tumors in children
    - • 50–60% of all spinal cord gliomas
    - • Localization in the ventricular system, mostly infratentorially, and spinal canal
    - • Well-circumscribed and gadolinium-enhancing on MRI
    - • 10 yr survival 45% in adults
    - • Total resection portends a better prognosis
  - − Anaplastic ependymoma (WHO grade III)
  - − Myxopapillary ependymoma (WHO grade I):
    - • Male: female ratio 2.2 : 1
    - • Occurs most frequently at the conus
    - • Associated with long-standing back pain
    - • Well-circumscribed and brightly gadolinium-enhancing on MRI
    - • Survival >10 yr with total (or partial) resection
  - − Subependymoma (WHO grade I):
    - • Often asymptomatic, found incidentally at autopsy
- ◆ Choroid plexus tumors:
  - − Choroid plexus papilloma (WHO grade I):
    - • Slow growing, benign
    - • Surgery usually curative
  - − Choroid plexus carcinoma (WHO grade III)
- ◆ Glial tumors of uncertain origin:
  - − Astroblastoma
  - − Gliomatosis cerebri
  - − Choroid glioma of third ventricle
- ◆ Neuronal and mixed neuronal-glial tumors:
  - − *See* WHO Classification reference for subtypes
- ◆ Neuroblastic tumors:
  - − Olfactory neuroblastoma
  - − Olfactory neuroepithelioma
  - − Neuroblastomas of the adrenal gland/sympathetic nervous system
- ◆ Pineal parenchymal tumors:
  - − Pineocytoma:
    - • Slow growing, usually favorable prognosis
  - − Pineoblastoma:
    - • Malignant, embryonal neoplasm
    - • Metastasizes via cerebrospinal fluid (CSF) pathways

    – Pineal parenchymal tumor of intermediate differentiation
- Embryonal tumors:
  - Medulloepiothelioma
  - Ependymoblastoma
  - Medulloblastoma
  - Supratentorial primitive neuroectodermal tumor
  - Atypical teratoid/rhabdoid tumor

Tumors of the Cranial and Peripheral Nerves

- Schwannoma (WHO grade I):
  - 8% of intracranial and 29% of spinal tumors
  - Occur mostly in the 4th–6th decade
  - Female: male ratio 2:1
  - Well-circumscribed, gadolinium-enhancing on MRI
  - Favorable prognosis, malignant change is exceedingly rare
- Neurofibroma (WHO grade I):
  - Associated with neurofibromatosis type 1 (NF1):
- Perineuroma
- Malignant peripheral nerve sheath tumor (WHO grade III or IV):
  - Half of the cases occur in patients with NF1
  - 34% 5-yr survival, 23% 10-yr survival

Tumors of the Meninges

- Menigothelial cell tumors:
  - Meningioma:
    - Majority are benign (WHO grade I)
    - Several subtypes are aggressive (WHO grade II):
      - Atypical
      - Clear cell
      - Choroid
      - Rhabdoid
      - Papillary
      - Anaplastic
    - Occur in the sixth to seventh decade
    - Female: male ratio 3:2 except in hereditary meningiomas, where the ratio is equal
    - Common sites:
      - Cerebral convexities
      - Falx
      - Olfactory groove (may present with Foster–Kennedy syndrome: Anosmia, ipsilateral optic atrophy, contralateral papilledema)

□ Sphenoid ridge
□ Parasellar
□ Tentorium cerebelli
• May be calcified on imaging. Gadolinium-enhancing
on MRI
• Dural-based, frequently with a "dural tail"
• Extent of resection predicts the likelihood of recurrence (i.e.,
recurrence rates decrease with complete resection)
♦ Mesenchymal, nonmeningothelial:
– *See* WHO Classification reference for subtypes
♦ Primary melanocytic:
– *See* WHO Classification reference for subtypes
♦ Uncertain histiogenesis:
– Haemangioblastoma:
• Associated with Von Hippel–Lindau Disease

Lymphomas/Haematopoietic Neoplasms

♦ Malignant lymphoma:
– 6% of primary central nervous sytem (CNS) tumors in
immunocompetent and immunocompromised patients, lesions may
be multiple in immunocompromised patients
– Recent increasing incidence is due primarily to the increase in
the number of Acquired Immunodeficiency Syndrome (AIDS)
patients
– 98% of primary CNS lymphomas are B-cell lymphomas
– Tissue from 95% of immunocompromised patients with CNS
lymphoma shows Epstein–Barr virus DNA
– Supratentorial location in 60%
– Ocular and leptomeningeal involvement can occur
– Diffuse gadolinium enhancement on MRI
– Thalium-201-SPECT or FDG-PET used to differentiate from
toxoplasmosis in AIDS patients
– Steroids may render tissue diagnosis difficult, therefore should
not be started until after biopsy, unless clinically necessary
– Therapy involves chemotherapy and radiation
– Median survival 17–45 mo (immunocompetent), 2–6 mo
(immunocompromised)
– Prognosis is favorable with a solitary mass, younger age, high
functional status
♦ Plasmacytoma
♦ Granulocytic sarcoma

Germ Cell Tumors

♦ Germinoma
♦ Embryonal carcinoma
♦ Yolk sac tumors
♦ Choricarcinoma
♦ Teratoma
♦ Mixed germ cell tumors

Tumors of the Sellar Region

♦ Pituitary adenoma:
  – 10% of intracranial tumors
  – Arise from the adenohypophysis
  – Secreting or nonsecreting
  – Secreting tumors present with endocrine dysfunction:
    • Cushing's (adrenocorticotropic hormone excess)
    • Amenorrhea, galactorrhea (prolactin excess)
    • Acromegaly (growth hormone excess)
  – Nonsecreting tumors present with mass effect (e.g., visual loss)
  – Both secreting and nonsecreting tumors can cause panhypopituitarism
  – Evaluation:
    • Visual fields
    • Endocrine axis (*see* Box 1)
  – Transphenoidal approach is favored
  – Post-operative course may be complicated by pituitary hypofunction
  – Recurrence 12%, 4–8 yr postoperatively
♦ Craniopharyngioma
♦ Granular cell tumor

Metastatic Brain Tumors

♦ 26% of all brain tumors
♦ Most metastases occur at the gray-white junction
♦ 80% are supratentorial, 15% occur in the cerebellum
♦ 30–50% of metastases are solitary
♦ Gadolinium-enhancing on MRI, usually with a large amount of surrounding edema
♦ Origin:
  – Respiratory tract 50%
  – Breast 15%

**Box 1
Evaluation of the Endocrine Axis
in Patients With Pituitary Masses**

♦ Random cortisol level (Cortrosyn stimulation test if low)
♦ Thyroid stimulating hormone level and thyroid function panel
♦ Prolactin level (1.4–24 µg/L)
♦ Follicle stimulating hormone, luteinizing hormone and estradiol
or testosterone
♦ Insulin growth factor-1
♦ Fasting blood glucose

  – Skin/melanoma 10.5%
  – Unknown primary 11%
♦ Contrast-enhanced CT of the chest, abdomen, and pelvis, as well as
mammography, constitute the initial evaluation for the primary tumor

Specific Symptoms and Signs by Anatomic Location
Posterior Fossa

♦ More likely to present with signs and symptoms of elevated ICP
(headache, nausea, vomiting, papilledema)
♦ More common in children

Supratentorial

♦ More likely to present with seizures, focal neurologic deficits, and
symptoms of increased ICP
♦ More common in adults

Pituitary

♦ May result in endocrine dysfunction, visual disturbances, or pituitary apoplexy

Cerebellopontine Angle

♦ Cranial nerve (CN) VIII compression:
  – Sensorineural hearing loss
  – Tinnitus
  – Dysequilibrium
♦ CN VII compression:
  – Peripheral-type facial palsy

♦ CN V compression:
  – Facial numbness
  – Neuralgia and accompanying dysasthesias
♦ Involvement of brain stem and lower cranial nerves as tumor enlarges:
  – Ataxia, diplopia, nausea, vomiting, headache, vertigo
  – Hoarseness, dysphagia

Imaging of Brain Tumors

♦ CT with contrast
♦ MRI
  – More sensitive than head CT with contrast, especially for detecting multiple lesions, e.g., metastases
  – May be used for grading some tumors (e.g., in astrocytic tumors the presence of ring enhancement implies a higher grade)
♦ Cerebral angiography
  – Not routinely used for brain mass unless a vascular malformation is suspected
  – May see vascular "blush" with a meningioma

Tissue Diagnosis

♦ Stereotactic biopsy
♦ Open biopsy

Treatment

Primary Treatment

♦ Surgical resection:
  – Total resection
  – Subtotal resection (debulking)
♦ Systemic chemotherapy (choice made based on tumor type)
♦ Implantable chemotherapeutic wafers (usually reserved for high-grade glial tumors)
♦ Local- or whole-brain radiation therapy (used mostly in high-grade lesions, in cases of multiple metastases, and radio-sensitive tumors)

Treatment of Seizures

♦ Phenytoin:
  – 15–20 mg/kg IV load, no faster than 50 mg/min. Target level 10–20 µg/mL
  – Alternatively, fosphenytoin can be used, especially in the elderly:
    • Dose: 15–20 mg/kg phenytoin equivalents
    • Route: IV or IM

♦ Common alternatives to IV phenytoin:
  – Valproic acid (target level 50–150 (μg/mL) or phenobarbitol
  (target level 25–40 μg/mL):
    • 15–20 mg/kg IV load

Treatment of Mass/Edema

♦ Dexamethasone. Tumor-associated vasogenic edema is highly sensitive to corticosteroids:
  – 4–10 mg PO/IV q 6 h.
♦ Optimize serum sodium, maintain normonatremia
♦ Use hypertonic saline or mannitol as needed for mass effect and impending herniation (*see* Chapter 5), as a bridge to surgery

Treatment of Hydrocephalus

♦ Intraventricular catheter for externalized CSF drainage. High risk of herniation with intracranial compartmental shifts and elevated ICP secondary to tumor. Use as a bridge to shunt
♦ Ventriculoperitoneal shunt:
  – Concerns include "seeding" of tumor cells to the peritoneum and occlusion by high CSF protein

Treatment of Endocrine Dysfunction

♦ As indicated by the results of endocrine axis evaluation (e.g., bromocriptine can be used to shrink prolactin-secreting tumors and normalize prolactin levels)

Treatment of Pituitary Apoplexy

♦ Stress dose steroids
♦ Evaluation of the endocrine axis
♦ Emergent decompression in case of visual loss or neurologic deterioration

Postoperative Management in the Intensive Care Unit (*see* Chapter 7)

♦ Frequent neurological examinations and STAT evaluation of any changes (*see* Box 2)
♦ Monitoring for signs of pituitary hypofunction (e.g., diabetes insipidus) in patients who had pituitary surgery
♦ Maintenance of appropriate antiepileptic drug levels in patients with seizures or at increased risk for seizures

♦ Maintenance of a normal metabolic milieu, most importantly normonatremia, normoglycemia, and euthermia

Routine Post-Operative Evaluation

♦ MRI with gadolinium to evaluate the operative bed for residual tumor, usually on the day after surgery

Prognosis

Primary Brain Tumors

♦ Depends primarily on pathological tumor grade

Metastatic Tumors

♦ Better prognosis:
  - Younger patients
  - Solitary lesion
  - Favorable location of lesions
  - High sensitivity to chemo- or radio-therapy
  - Favorable behavior of the primary tumor

Key Points

♦ Clinical presentation depends on tumor location. Factors affecting the clinical presentation include the presence of elevated ICP and/or hydrocephalus, as well as pituitary (endocrine dysfunction), cranial nerve (cranial nerve palsies), and cortical (seizures) involvement

♦ Treatment is individualized, taking into account the location, type, grade of tumor, as well as general patient characteristics. The main treatment modalities include resection, steroids, chemotherapy, and radiation

♦ Prognosis for primary brain tumors depends largely on pathological tumor grade

♦ Immediate postoperative management focuses on judicious monitoring of the neurologic exam, maintenance of a normal metabolic milieu, maintenance of therapeutic antiepileptic drug levels, and monitoring for complications (e.g., diabetes insipidus in pituitary tumor resection)

Suggested Reading

Kleihues, P and Cavenee, WK, eds. World Health Organization Classification of Tumours, Pathology and Genetics, *Tumours of the Nervous System,* Lyon, France: IARC; 2000.

Greenberg, MS. *Handbook of Neurosurgery,* Lakeland, FL: Greenberg Graphics, Inc.; 1997.

Bradley, WG, Daroff, RB, Fenichel, GM, and Marsden, CD. *Neurology in Clinical Practice: Principles of Diagnosis and Management,* Woburn, MA: Butterworth-Heinemann; 2000:1235–1309.

11 Hydrocephalus

Geoffrey S. F. Ling

Hydrocephalus

♦ Defined as dilation of cerebral ventricles

Types

♦ Communicating
♦ Noncommunicating
♦ Hydrocephalus ex vacuole
♦ Other:
  – Arrested hydrocephalus
  – Normal pressure hydrocephalus
  – Hydrocephalus ex vacuole

Cerebrospinal fluid

♦ Anatomy:
  – Formed by combined processes of diffusion, active transport, and free water passage
  – Cerebrospinal fluid (CSF) is produced mainly by choroid plexus, which reside in the cerebral ventricles, third and fourth ventricles. Other sites of production are the ependyma and, to a lesser degree, cerebral pial surface
  – Beginning in the two lateral cerebral ventricles (left and right), CSF flows, under hydrostatic pressure, through the interventricular foramen (formen of Monro) and into the third ventricle, then along the aqueduct of Sylvius into the fourth ventricle and finally exits via the centrally located foramen of Magendie and two lateral foramina of Luschka into the cisterna magna and subarachnoid space

From: *Current Clinical Neurology: Handbook of Neurocritical Care*
Edited by: A. Bhardwaj, M. A. Mirski, and J. A. Ulatowski © Humana Press Inc., Totowa, NJ

- While in the subarachnoid space, CSF bathes the entire central nervous system, nerve roots, and central canal of the spinal cord
- CSF is eventually resorbed through arachnoid granulations or villi in the superior sagittal sinus into the venous system
♦ CSF is formed at a rate of 0.3 cc/min or 20 cc/hr
♦ Total CSF volume is approx 150 cc with 75 cc in the cranial vault
♦ CSF is under intracranial pressure (ICP), which is normally approx 10 mmHg
♦ CSF is normally clear, colorless, acellular (up to 5 white blood cells [wbc]/mm³), protein 15–45 mg/dL, glucose 2/3 blood glucose and sterile

Causes of Hydrocephalus

♦ Communicating:
  - CSF is able to exit the ventricular system
  - The basis of this condition is obstruction of CSF resorption at the level of the arachnoid villi
  - This is also referred to as extraventricular obstructive hydrocephalus (EVOH)
  - Caused by obstruction of arachnoid granulations
  - Conditions:
    • Vascular: Subarachnoid hemorrhage (SAH), intraventricular hemorrhage (IVH)
    • Infectious: Fungal, bacterial, less commonly viral
♦ Noncommunicating:
  - CSF is unable to exit the ventricular system
  - There is obstruction within the ventricular system leading to trapped CSF
  - Also known as intraventricular obstructive hydrocephalus (IVOH)
  - Frequently caused by obstruction at outflow tract (e.g., fourth ventricle, third ventricle, or interventricular foraminae)
  - Conditions:
    • Hemorrhage: IVH
    • Tumor
    • Edema
    • Inflammation
♦ Hydrocephalus ex vacuole:
  - Enlargement of ventricles as a result of cerebral atrophy
  - Conditions:
    • Aging
    • Neurodegenerative conditions
    • Alzheimer's disease

♦ Other:
  – Normal pressure hydrocephalus (NPH)
  – Arrested hydrocephalus

Diagnosis

♦ Symptoms:
  – Often subtle initially:
    • Headache: Usually mild
    • Visual changes
    • Gait disturbance, including ataxia and apraxia
    • Seizure
  – Change in mental status:
    • Encephalopathy, including both acute confusional state and dementia
    • Decreased level of consciousness
    • Chronically, may be more subcortical in nature
  – If ICP is increased, nausea and vomiting
♦ Signs:
  – If ICP is increased, then papilledema
  – Neurologic exam may be normal or nonfocal
  – For normal pressure hydrocephalus, there is the classic triad of dementia, ataxia, and urinary incontinence
♦ Diagnostic studies:
  – Neuroimaging:
    • CT-head noncontrast
    • MRI with T1 and T2 imaging
  – CT findings:
    • Dilated cerebral ventricles
    • Bowing of third ventricle if under pressure
    • Fourth ventricle is dilated in communicating hydrocephalus
    • Absence of fourth ventricular dilation is suggestive of non-communicating hydrocephalus
  – MRI findings:
    • Dilated ventricles
    • Increased T2-weighted signal in periventricular area signifying transependymal CSF flow
  – Radioisotope cisternography:
    • Injection of radioisotope into the lumbar thecal sac
    • If there is reflux, isotope will appear in the ventricles
    • Normally, isotope distributes over the cerebral convexities

– Lumbar puncture (LP):
  • Cerebrospinal fluid: normal
  • Opening pressure: may be increased
  • LP should be avoided when noncommunicating hydro-cephalus is present

Treatment

♦ If communicating, serial LPs
♦ Consider trial of large volume (40–60 cc) CSF drainage
♦ Consider trial of lumbar drain
♦ If noncommunicating, intraventricular catheter (IVC)
♦ Lumbar drain:
  – Volume directed: remove 10 cc/h for 2–3 d
  – Pressure directed: place drain at pop-off of 10 mmHg for 2–3 d
  – Pressure-volume directed: every hour, remove enough CSF to achieve ICP of 10mmHg. Continue for 2–3 d
♦ Intraventricular catheter:
  – Initially place drain pop-off at 0 mmHg. This will allow external drainage of all CSF (i.e., 20 cc/h)
  – An added benefit is that in cases of IVH, blood products will be removed from the ventricular system
  – As the patient clinically improves, the pop-off may be increased. Initially, it should be to 5 or 10 mmHg. If the CSF drainage exceeds 10 cc/h, then the ICP is greater than the pop-off. There may also be ICP waves. Some ICP waves are pathologic, such as A or plateau waves. Indicative of poor brain compliance. However, if the CSF drainage is <10 cc/hr and the patient has not neurologically deteriorated, then a higher pop-off may be considered. Once a patient has been shown to tolerate a pop-off of 20 mm Hg, then a trial of monitoring only (i.e., no CSF drainage) should be attempted prior to IVC removal
♦ Shunt:
  – If a patient cannot tolerate increasing pop-off, one should consider an indwelling shunt system.
  – Disqualifying criteria are persistent blood products, high protein (>300mg/dL) or infection
  – For NPH, if a patient improves with CSF drainage, then one can consider placing an indwelling shunt system
  – Systems are generally either ventricle to peritoneal (VP) or lumbar to peritoneal (LP). Others that are less common are VJ (ventricle to jugular) or VA (ventricle to cardiac atrium)

Complications

◆ Subdural hematoma:
  – Rapid or over decompression of ventricles may lead to retraction of atrophic brain from inner calvarial table causing tearing of bridging veins
  – If severe, it may necessitate surgical drainage
◆ Infection may develop, especially during external drainage. Thus, when using an IVC or lumbar drain, prophylactic antibiotics are indicated. Usually Gram-positive coverage with oxacillin or clindamycin (if pencillin allergy) is adequate. Surveillance CSF specimens should be collected sterilely every day or two from the drainage system for CSF analysis (cells and type, protein, glucose, Gram stain, and culture). Evidence of infection should result in removing the drain and placing a new one in a new location

Key Points

◆ Hydrocephalus is a common accompaniment of acute brain injury
◆ Communicating vs noncommunicating hydrocephalus must be distinguished by neuroimaging techniques
◆ External CSF drainage can be life-saving in acute obstructive hydrocephalus
◆ Infectious complications are the most common with IVC

Suggested Reading

Afifi A. and Bergman R. *Functional Neuroanatomy: Text and Atlas,* New York: McGraw-Hill; 1998.

Ariada N and Sotelo J. Review: treatment of hydrocephalus in adults, *Surg Neuro* 2002;58:377–384.

Suarez-Rivera O. Acute hydrocephalus after subarachnoid hemorrhage. *Surg Neuro* 1998;49: 563–565.

McAllister JP. Hydrocephalus enters the new millennium: an overview. *Neurol Res* 2000;22:2–3.

Pattisapu J. Etiology and clinical course of hydrocephalus. *Neurosurg Clin N Amer* 2001;12:651–659.

Bradley WG. Diagnostic tools in hydrocephalus. *Neruosurg Clin N Amer* 2001;12:661–684.

12   Spinal Cord Injury

Robert D. Stevens

Epidemiology

♦ Demographics (in the United States):
  - Common causes of acute spinal cord injury (SCI) (Table 1):
    • Trauma (most common)
    • Degenerative spine disease
    • Ischemia, demyelination
    • Inflammation
    • Rapidly expanding neoplastic, hemorrhagic, or pyogenic masses
  - Traumatic SCI has an incidence of 28–55 million/yr, prevalence is 200,000, male to female ratio is 4:1, and average age 32 yr. Traumatic SCI is most frequently secondary to:
    • Motor vehicle accidents (40–50%)
    • Assault (10–25%)
    • Falls (20%)
    • Work-related (10–25%).
  - Cervical spine involved in 55% of traumatic SCI
  - Acute nontraumatic spinal cord compression most commonly is in the thoracic region
♦ Outcome:
  - Three month mortality after SCI is approx 30%
  - Predictors of mortality are level of cord injury, Glasgow Coma Scale (GCS), and respiratory failure
  - Leading causes of death after SCI:
    • Respiratory failure
    • Cardiovascular insufficiency
    • Pulmonary embolism

From: *Current Clinical Neurology: Handbook of Neurocritical Care*
Edited by: A. Bhardwaj, M. A. Mirski, and J. A. Ulatowski © Humana Press Inc., Totowa, NJ

Table 1
Causes of Spinal Cord Injury

Traumatic
Rheumatological
  Spondylosis
  Intervertebral disc herniation
Neoplastic
  Metastatic
  Primary
Infectious
  Pyogenic (epidural abscess)
  Tuberculosis (Pott's disease)
  Viral (poliovirus, VZV, HSV, CMV, HIV, HTLV-1)
  Spirochetal (Lyme disease, syphilis)
  Parasitic (Toxoplasma, Schistosoma)
Inflammatory-immune
  Multiple sclerosis
  Trasverse myelitis
  Postinfectious myelitis
  Paraneoplastic myelitis
  Sarcoidosis
Vascular
  Spinal cord infarction
  Hemorrhage/hematoma (epidural, subdural, hematomyelia)
  Arteriovenous malformation
Toxic/metabolic
  Chemotherapeutic agents
  Radiation
  Subacute combined degeneration (vitamin B_{12} deficiency)

- Sepsis
- Suicide
– 10–15% of patients with complete SCI achieve some degree of functional recovery; 54–86% with incomplete SCI achieve some functional recovery

Pathogenesis

♦ Anatomy:
  – Transverse section of spinal cord reveals central "H-shaped" gray matter and surrounding white matter tracts. Of the many white matter tracts, only three can be assessed by physical examination:
    • Anterolateral spinothalamic tract: pain, temperature, light touch, and pressure
    • Posterolateral corticospinal tract: motor commands.
    • Posterior columns: fine touch, vibration, and position sense
  – White matter tracts organized somatotopically, cervical fibers medial, thoracic fibers intermediate, lumbosacral fibers more lateral
  – Cord blood supply is from one anterior spinal (anterior two thirds of cord) and two posterior spinal (posterior one third of cord) arteries, branches of the vertebrals. Thyrocervical, costocervical, intercostals, and lumbar arteries provide additional blood flow in thoracolumbar segments. Risk of watershed infarcts at boundaries between anterior/posterior and cervical/thoracic or thoracic/lumbar territories
♦ Vascular physiology:
  – Spinal cord blood flow (SCBF) is regulated analogously to cerebral blood flow (CBF):
    • Average 50 mL/100 g/min
    • Autoregulation between a mean arterial pressure of 60 and 150
    • Increases with hypercapnia and severe hypoxemia
  – Spinal cord perfusion is also dependent on intrathecal pressure and may be ameliorated by cerebrospinal fluid (CSF) drainage
  – Traumatic SCI impairs SCBF autoregulation
♦ Pathophysiology:
  – SCI is the result of primary and secondary injury mechanisms:
    • Primary injury: damage incurred during initial insult, maximal at onset, unlikely to be modified by therapeutic intervention
    • Secondary injury: may be significantly influenced by systemic factors such as blood pressure, cardiac output, oxygenation. Abnormalities include:

□ Vascular impairment: increased permeability, vasospasm, thrombosis, and hemorrhage

□ Inflammatory changes: local and systemic mediator release, expression of cell adhesion molecules, and leukocyte infiltration

□ Cellular dysfunction: adenosine triphosphate (ATP) depletion, plasma membrane failure, free radical generation, excitatory amino acid release, cellular calcium overload, and mitochondrial insufficiency

– Beyond these acute changes, injurious mechanisms may continue to unfold with delayed cell death, glial scar, and cystic cavity formation

Diagnosis

♦ Clinical assessment:

– Initial concerns:

• Adequacy of airway, breathing, and circulatory function

• Presence of associated injuries:

□ 25–50% of patients with traumatic SCI have traumatic brain injury (TBI)

□ 5–10% of patients with TBI have SCI

□ Truncal injuries in 10–20% of patients with thoracic or lumbar SCI

□ Noncontiguous spine injury in 10% of patients with cervical spine injury

• Physical examination should include inspection for spinal deformity, palpation for deformity or tenderness, motor (including sphincter) function, sensory function, and deep tendon reflexes.

– *Neurologic level.* Most caudal segment with bilateral normal motor (antigravity strength ≥ 3/5) and sensory (light touch and pinprick) sensation

– *Complete injury* signifies abolition of all motor and sensory function below the lesion. The *zone of partial preservation* is an area adjacent to the neurologic level in which there are abnormal sensory or motor findings. An area of abnormal findings that is not contiguous with the postulated level qualifies as incomplete injury and would mandate a reassessment of the level

– *Spinal shock* is characterized by flaccid arreflexic paralysis and anaesthesia to all modalities. Present in one half of SCI patients, it has a variable time course but resolves in less than 24 h in >90% of cases. Should be distinguished from neurogenic shock (below)

Table 2
ASIA Impairment Scale

Grade	Description	Incidence	Outcome
A	Complete motor and sensory loss	25%	10–15% convert to grades B–C; 3% to grade D
B	Incomplete sensory loss, complete motor loss	15%	54% convert to grade C–D
C	Incomplete motor and sensory loss; more than 50% of muscles < 3/5	10%	86% of grades C–D eventually regain ambulating
D	Incomplete motor and sensory loss; more than 50% of muscles ≥ 3/5	30%	ability
E	Normal motor and sensory function		

ASIA, American Spinal Injury Association.

– The widely used American Spine Injury Association (ASIA) clinical scoring system records motor strength in 10 muscle groups and sensory function in 28 dermatomes. The ASIA impairment scale combines severity of deficits with completeness of injury and is predictive of outcome (*see* Table 2)
– Spinal cord syndromes based on anatomic localization are detailed in Table 3
♦ Imaging:
– Goal of imaging is identify rapidly injury of the spine that places neural tissue at risk
– When all radiographic modalities (standard radiographs, computerized tomography [CT], and magnetic resonance imaging [MRI]) are combined, greater than 95% of patients with traumatic SCI are found to have associated spine injury. Spinal cord injury without radiographic abnormality (SCIWORA) refers to a subgroup of patients with cord-induced deficits who have no detectable changes on plain radiographs or CT
– Imaging should be obtained in all trauma patients with risk factors for cord or spine injury (*see* Table 4)
– Standard cervical radiographs include anteroposterior, lateral, and odontoid views. Technically adequate films allow visualiza-

Table 3
Spinal Cord Syndromes

Syndrome	Setting	Clinical findings
Complete cord (cord transection)	Trauma, infarction, hemorrhage, disc herniation, transverse myelitis, tumor, abscess	Loss of all motor and sensory function. Cord transection above C3 results in apnea and death unless prompt recuscitation
Brown–Sequard (cord hemisection)	Penetrating trauma, multiple sclerosis, tumor, abscess	Ipsilateral loss of proprioception and motor function. Contralateral pain and temperature loss. Suspended ipsilateral loss of all sensory modalities
Central cord	Neck hyperextension, syringomyelia, intramedullary tumor	Motor impairment greater in upper than lower extremity. Suspended sensory loss in cervicothoracic dermatomes
Anterior cord	Hyperflexion, disc protrusion, anterior spinal artery occlusion	Pain and temperature loss with sparing of proprioception. Variable motor impairment
Posterior cord	Classically, syphilis, vitamin B12 deficiency; more commonly, multiple sclerosis	Diminished proprioception and fine touch
Conus medullaris	Tumor, trauma, disc herniation, inflammation, infection	Extension to lumbosacral roots may produce both upper and lower motor neuron signs. Spastic paraparesis, sphincter dysfunction, lower sacral "saddle" sensory loss
Cauda equina[a]	Herniated disc, spinal stenosis, inflammation, infection, intrathecal lidocaine, continuous spinal anesthesia microcatheters	Sensory changes in a saddle distribution; lower back pain; sciatica; bowel and bladder dysfunction; variable motor loss in lower extremities

[a]Not a myelopathy but a radiculopathy or neuropathy involving lumbosacral nerves.

Table 4
Risk Factors for Spine or Spinal Cord Injury in Trauma Patients

Neck or back pain or tenderness
Sensory or motor deficits
Impaired level of consciousness
Alcohol or drug intoxication
Painful, distracting injuries outside the spine/spinal cord region

tion of the entire cervical spine to the C7-T1 intervetebral space. Lateral views should be screened for changes in vertebral alignment, bony structure, intervetebral space, and soft tissue
  – Flexion-extension views. Useful for detecting occult instability resulting from ligamentous injury. Safe only in patients who are neurologically intact, not intoxicated, and in whom there is no subluxation >3.5 mm on lateral films
  – CT:
    • Indications:
      □ Spine is not adequately visualized or appears abnormal on standard films
      □ Clinical suspicion is high in spite of normal, technically adequate standard films
    • Negative predictive value of normal, technically adequate standard films combined with CT is >99%
  – MR is highly sensitive to nonosseous changes including spinal cord edema, hemorrhage, and ligamentous injury. MRI is indicated in the presence of any cord-related neurologic findings. For bony trauma, CT may be more sensitive
♦ Spinal stability:
  – Defined as the capacity of the spine to withstand physiologic loading without neurologic injury, deformity, or pain. Predicted based on clinical and imaging characteristics. For thoracolumbar spine, CT-based three column model is frequently used (instability defined as injury to more than two columns):
    • Anterior column: Anterior longitudinal ligament, anterior half of vertebral body or disc
    • Middle column: Posterior half of body or disc and posterior longitudinal ligament
    • Posterior column: Posterior arch and ligaments

- Clearing (establishing stability) of the cervical spine in trauma
patients. Initial trauma management assumes that the spine is
unstable until proven otherwise:
  • All trauma patients should be screened for clinical risk factors of spine or cord injury (*see* Table 4). When all five of these
  factors are absent, cervical spine injury may be ruled out by
  clinical examination with a negative predictive value of >99%:
  after removing immobilizing device, active and passive neck
  movement should be painless and elicit no neurologic symptoms
  • Patients with risk factors should have three view plain radiographs and CT if plain films are abnormal or inadequate
  • Patients with neurologic deficits ascribable to cord injury
  should undergo MRI

Management in the Intensive Care Unit

♦ Traumatic SCI is frequently associated with brain injury and with
alterations in respiratory and cardiovascular function that require critical care management. Specific complications include respiratory failure, atelectasis, pneumonia, neurogenic shock, autonomic dysreflexia,
venous thromboembolism, and sepsis. Critical care management
goals include:
  – Maximizing chances of neurologic recovery by limiting secondary injury mechanisms
  – Providing supportive care for systemic repercussions and complications of SCI
♦ Immobilization:
  – Goal is to prevent neurologic injury in the presence of an unstable spine
  – Should include the whole spine until lumbar and thoracic injury
  are ruled out by physical examination and imaging
  – Complications of immobilization: Pain, decubitus ulcers, and
  impaired chest wall mobility in up to 70% of patients. May also
  increase risk of airway compromise, difficult intubation, aspiration, and increased intracranial pressure (ICP)
♦ Surgical management:
  – Goals are to decompress neural tissue, and to prevent spinal
  cord and nerve root injury by ensuring realignment and mechanical stability of the spine. Surgical options include:
    • Mechanical traction with cranial tongs or halo ring/vest.
    Contraindications include atlanto-occipital dissociation, types
    IIA or III hangman's fracture, and skull defect at anticipated
    pin insertion site

- Operative management. Generally includes reduction/decompression, and fixation.
  - In patients with cord compression and stable neurologic findings, it is unclear whether early (<24 h after injury) surgical intervention improves neurologic outcomes when compared to delayed surgery
  - Indications for early/emergent operative management:
    - Irreducible bilateral facet dislocation and incomplete tetraplegia
    - Rapidly deteriorating neurologic deficits
- ◆ Airway management:
  - Airway management in patients with spine or cord trauma is challenging:
    - Intubation has been linked to severe cord injury and death
    - Airway may be obstructed by concomitant face and neck injury, blood, vomitus, foreign bodies, edema, or retropharyngeal hematoma
  - Goal is to ensure rapid control of the airway while incurring minimal neurologic risk. Principle is to minimize neck movement during the procedure
  - Indications for intubation in patients with SCI:
    - Airway compromise: Edema, retropharyngeal hematoma, elevated aspiration risk
    - Respiratory failure:
      - □ Significant decline in forced vital capacity (FVC) or FVC <15 mL/kg
      - □ Increased work of breathing
      - □ PaO_2 < 60 mmHg or significant decline on supplemental oxygen
      - □ Primary respiratory acidosis with pH <7.25
    - Associated TBI:
      - □ GCS < 8
      - □ Intracranial hypertension
      - □ Herniation
  - Airway management techniques:
    - Blind nasotracheal intubation. May be useful in the field, however >20% failure rate
    - Direct laryngoscopy and endotracheal intubation with manual in-line stabilization. Preferred technique when the airway must be secured emergently, and/or in an uncooperative patient
    - Awake fiberoptic-guided intubation via the nasal or oral route. Preferred method for nonemergent intubation in cooperative patients

- Complications of airway management:
  - Cord injury. Thought to be rare in clinical practice, but documented in several case reports. Many experimental studies indicate significant displacement of spine during laryngoscopy. Establishing a causal relation between intubation and subsequent cord injury may be difficult because of confounding by post-intubation events which independently may have precipitated or potentiated SCI, including surgical manipulation, changes in position, hypotension and hypoxia
  - Hypotension may result from the negative inotropic and vasodilating effects of agents used for sedation, from the attenuation of sympathetic tone associated with resolution of hypoxia and hypercarbia, and from the hemodynamic effects of positive pressure ventilation. Hypotension should be aggressively preempted by fluid and vasopressor admistration
  - Succinylcholine has been linked to severe hyperkalemia and cardiac arrest in patients with SCI and is contraindicated >24 h after injury
♦ Respiratory management:
  - Patients with acute cervical SCI are at increased risk for respiratory failure and complications such as aspiration, atelectasis, pneumonia, pulmonary embolism, and acute respiratory distress syndrome (ARDS). Pulmonary complications are promoted by, and may exacerbate, underlying neurogenic ventilatory insufficiency, generating a spiral of deteriorating respiratory function
  - Respiratory failure is an independent predictor of short-term mortality and a leading cause of death in patients with SCI
  - Pathophysiology:
    - Cervical cord injury is associated with alterations in ventilatory control, breathing patterns, and respiratory mechanics
    - Clinically, recruitment of accessory muscles with inspiration results in expansion of the upper rib cage while the flaccid diaphragm ascends into the thoracic cavity, generating a "paradoxical" inward movement of the lower rib cage and abdominal wall
    - Lung volumes are significantly reduced, producing a clinical pattern of rapid shallow breathing and a restrictive defect on pulmonary function testing. Pulmonary and chest wall compliance are decreased, contributing to a greater work of breathing
    - Respiratory muscle weakness leads to alveloar hypoventilation and hypercapnic hypoxemic respiratory insufficiency

- Weakness of abdominal wall muscles impairs coughing, decreasing effective clearance of secretions, leading to mucus plugging and atelectasis
- Pulmonary edema developing in the setting of SCI must elicit consideration of several distinct pathologic processes:
  - Congestive heart failure may develop because of loss of sympathetic myocardial innervation, in particular if intravenous fluid resuscitation is overzealous
  - ARDS may result from associated pulmonary infection, aspiration, lung trauma, sepsis
  - Neurogenic pulmonary may be precipitated by SCI. Pathogenesis is incompletely understood but thought to involve transient increased sympathetic outflow and venous pulmonary hypertension with fluid extravasation
- Pattern of respiratory dysfunction depends on the level of injury:
  - Complete injury above C3 causes respiratory arrest and death unless immediate ventilatory assistance is given. Survivors need long-term ventilatory support or diaphragmatic pacing
  - Injury at the C3–C5 level leads to respiratory failure and the need for mechanical ventilation in the majority of patients
    - □ Onset of respiratory insufficiency is typically delayed, occurring on d 3–5 post-injury owing to rostral spread of cord edema
    - □ With the resolution of cord edema and spasticity of chest wall muscles, a progressive increase in lung volumes may be seen. Patients in this group generally recover sufficient ventilatory function to be liberated from the ventilator usually over a period of weeks
  - Injury below C5 is associated with a lesser degree of ventilatory failure. These patients remain at significant risk however for atelectasis and pneumonia
- Therapy for respiratory complications:
  - In animal and clinical paradigms of SCI, hypoxemia is associated with secondary injury and exacerbation of neurologic outcome
  - The majority of patients with significant cord injury above C5 will need mechanical ventilation. There is little data corre-

lating specific ventilator modes with respiratory outcomes and successful weaning
- When respiratory drive and diaphragmatic function are negligible, complete modes of support such as assist-control or controlled mandatory ventilation are required
- When residual drive and diaphragmatic function are present, interactive modes such as synchronized intermittent mandatory ventilation, pressure support ventilation, or combinations of these, may limit respiratory muscle deconditioning
- Atelectasis may be pre-empted and treated with positive end-expiratory pressure. Lobar atelectasis or complete lung collapse may require selective fiberoptic bronchoscopy to restore patency of occluded airways
- Risk of ventilator associated pneumonia increases with duration of mechanical ventilation and ultimately a significant proportion of patients with SCI will develop this complication. Risk may be decreased by maintaining head of bed at 30°
- Tracheostomy should be considered if mechanical ventilation is anticipated to last >2–3 wk

♦ Cardiovascular management:
   – Experimental evidence indicates that blood pressure autoregulation of SCBF is lost in SCI, as in TBI
   – *Neurogenic shock:*
      - Refers to a hemodynamic syndrome, to be distinguished from neurologic syndrome of spinal shock (above). More common when SCI is in upper thoracic or cervical segments
      - Suggested by a pattern of hypotension with an inappropriately normal or even low heart rate; it reflects sympathetic denervation of the heart (T1 to T4) and vasculature with resulting decreased inotropism, chronotropism, and arterial and venous dilation
      - Depending on the degree of myocardial impairment cardiac output may be decreased, normal or even increased, whereas systemic vascular resistance is invariably decreased
   – Therapeutic approach:
      - Hypotension and shock are associated with secondary injury and worsening of neurologic outcomes after SCI and must be aggressively prevented and corrected
      - Consideration should be given to all potential causes of hemodynamic instability including bleeding, tension pneumothorax, myocardial injury, pericardial tamponade, sepsis, and neurogenic shock

- Restrospective studies of patients with acute SCI suggest that hemodynamic support with volume expansion and/or blood pressure augmentation may be achieved safely and may be associated with better neurologic outcomes
- Hemodynamic instability mandates invasive monitoring including arterial and central venous canulation. If shock does not promptly resolve, pulmonary artery catheterization or echocardiographic assessment may provide useful insight
- Fluid resuscitation is necessary in most patients with SCI owing to diminished effective circulating volume (hemorrhage, inadequate fluid intake, and vasodilation). However, the aggressiveness of volume repletion must be balanced against the risk of precipitating congestive heart failure, in particular if myocardial sympathetic innervation is lost
- Pharmacologic support:
  - □ If there is evidence of cardiac dysfunction, an agent with significant inotropic and vasoconstrictive effects such as dopamine or epinephrine is recommended
  - □ If no significant cardiac dysfunction is present, a vasoconstrictor such as phenylephrine or noreprinephrine should be used
- Hemodynamic interventions should guided by explicit clinical and physiologic endpoints such as heart rate, cardiac output, urine output, and neurologic examination
- ◆ Venous thromboembolism:
  - – Patients with SCI incur the highest risk of venous thromboembolism of all hospitalized patients
  - – Deep venous thrombosis:
    - In SCI patients not receiving prophylaxis, 39–100% develop deep venous thrombosis
    - Among trauma patients, presence of spinal cord injury is the strongest predictor of DVT
    - Risk is higher with complete SCI, with thoracic SCI, and during the first 3 mo after injury
  - – Pulmonary embolism (PE) occurs in 4–10% of patients not receiving prophylaxis. It is one of the three leading causes of death after SCI
  - – Prevention:
    - Although definitive evidence is lacking, current guidelines from both the American Association of Neurologic Surgeons and the American College of Chest Physicians recommend that

patients with SCI receive prophylaxis with low-molecular-weight heparin or unfractionated heparin associated with mechanical compression devices

• Uncertainty remains as to how soon after injury prophylaxis may be safely instituted, and for how long it should be prolonged

• Vena cava filters have been advocated to prevent PE in this high-risk population. However, prospective clinical trials to support this practice are lacking. Filters should be considered in patients who fail heparin or hirudin therapy or who present significant contraindications to anticoagulation

♦ Corticosteroids:

– Experimentally, corticosteroids attenuate inflammatory changes, edema, lipid peroxidation, excitotoxicity and cytoskeletal degradation associated with SCI

– High-dose methylprednisolone sulfate (MPSS) was evaluated in several large randomized trials of SCI patients:

• In National Acute Spinal Cord Injury Study II (NASCIS II), published in 1990, MPSS had no effect on neurologic outcome when compared to naloxone or placebo. However post-hoc subgroup analysis revealed that patients receiving the drug <8 h after injury had better motor scores at 6 mo and 1 yr when compared to those receiving MPSS at later timepoints

• In NASCIS III, published in 1997, MPSS given for 48 h was no better than MPSS given for 23 h or than tirilazad given for 48 h. Again, a post-hoc assessment showed that among patients treated 3–8 h after injury, 48 h of MPSS was associated with better motor scores at 6 wk and 6 mo than 23 h of the drug.

• In both studies, use of MPSS was associated with a higher risk of infectious complications

– Based on these results, MPSS has entered into widespread clinical practice and is regarded as a standard of care by many clinicians. However, the original studies have been come under increasing scrutiny for serious methodologic flaws and the clinical role of MPSS and other corticosteroids in patients with SCI is being actively questioned

– Dosing regimens based on NASCIS II and III:

• For SCI <3 h: MPSS 30 mg/kg IV, then 5.4 mg/kg/h for 23 h

• For SCI 3–8 h: MPSS 30 mg/kg IV, then 5.4 mg/kg/h for 48 h

♦ Other issues:
  – Infection. Patients with acute SCI are at increased risk for infectious complications, and sepsis is a leading cause of death in this patient population. The most common infections are pulmonary and urinary tract infections. Fever without an evident source may be caused by occult peritonitis that may develop insidiously without pain or guarding and should be assessed for with appropriate imaging
  – Gastrointestinal. Gastroparesis and paralytic ileus are common after SCI and may increase risk of aspiration. Metoclopramide or erythromycin may useful in this setting
  – Autonomic dysreflexia refers to a syndrome of paroxysmal hypertension, bradycardia, and headache that develops in response to a stimulus below the level of cord injury:
    • Occurs in up to 70–90% of patients with a lesion above T6, typically beginning weeks to months after the original insult. Common precipitants include distension of viscera and surgical stimulation. If untreated, may lead to stroke, intracerebral hemorrhage, dysrhythmias, myocardial infarction, and congestive heart failure
    • Treatment:
      □ Identify and remove the precipitating stimulus
      □ Administer vasodilators (hydralazine, nitroprusside, nicardipine)

Key Points (Table 5)

♦ Acute traumatic SCI is commonly associated with brain injury and other organ dysfunction requiring critical care management
♦ Complications of SCI include respiratory failure, atelectasis, pneumonia, neurogenic shock, autonomic dysreflexia, venous thromboembolism, and sepsis
♦ Acute care management should be directed to minimizing secondary injury by optimizing cord perfusion and oxygenation with the appropriate level of hemodynamic and respiratory support
♦ Methylprednisolone, when instituted less than 8 h after traumatic SCI, was associated in two clinical trials with statistically significant increments in motor scores at six months and one year. However, the clinical relevance of these data are uncertain

Table 5
Critical Care Issues in Spinal Cord Injury

System	Problem	Management
Neurologic	Secondary injury	Immobilization
		Surgical decompression
		Adequate perfusion and oxygenation
		Corticosteroids
Cardiovascular	Neurogenic shock	Invasive monitoring
		Volume resuscitation
		Vasopressor agents
		Inotropic agents
	Autonomic dysreflexia	Removal of stimulus
		Vasodilators
Hemostasis	Deep venous thrombosis	LMWH prophylaxis
	Pulmonary embolism	Therapeutic heparin
		Vena cava filter
Respiratory	Ventilatory failure	Mechanical ventilation
		Tracheostomy
	Pneumonia	Antimicrobial therapy
	Atelectasis	Incentive spirometry, PEEP
Gastrointestinal	Stress ulcer	H2-blocker prophylaxis
	Gastroparesis, paralytic ileus	Metoclopramide, erythromycin
	Occult peritonitis	Surgery, antimicrobials
Urinary	Urinary tract infection	Antimicrobials
Skin	Decubitus ulcers	Prevention protocols
		Wound care
		Plastic and reconstructive surgery
Psychiatric	Anxiety	Sedation, pain control
	Depression	Counseling
	Suicide	

LMWH, low molecular weight heparin; PPI, proton-pump inhibitor.

Suggested Reading

Amar AP and Levy ML. Surgical controversies in the management of spinal cord injury. *J Am Coll Surg* 1999;188:550–566

Bracken MB, Shepard MJ, Collins WF, et al. A randomized, controlled trial of methylprednisolone or naloxone in the treatment of acute spinal-cord injury: results of the second national acute spinal cord injury study. *N Engl J Med* 1990;322:1405–1411.

Bracken MB, Shepard MJ, Holford TR, et al. Administration of methyl-prednisolone for 24 or 48 h or tirilazad mesylate for 48 h in the treatment of acute spinal cord injury. *JAMA* 1997;277:1597–1604.

Geerts WH, Heit JA, Clagett GP, et al. Prevention of venous thromboembolism. *Chest* 2001;119:132S–175S

Guidelines of the American Association of Neurologic Surgeons and the Congress of Neurologic Surgeons. Pharmacological therapy after cervical spinal cord injury. *Neurosurgery* 2002;50:S63–S67

Guidelines of the American Association of Neurologic Surgeons and the Congress of Neurologic Surgeons. Radiographic assessment of the cervical spine in symptomatic trauma patients. *Neurosurgery* 2002;50:S36–S43

Guidelines of the American Association of Neurologic Surgeons and the Congress of Neurologic Surgeons. Radiographic assessment of the cervical spine in aymptomatic trauma patients. *Neurosurgery* 2002;50:S30–S35

Hoffman JR, Mower WR, Wolfson AB, et al. Validity of a set of clinical criteria to rule out injury to the cervical spine in patients with blunt trauma. National Emergency X-Radiography Utilization. Study Group. *N Engl J Med* 2000 Jul 13;343(2):94–99.

Hurlbert RJ. The role of steroids in acute spinal cord injury. An evidence-based analysis. *Spine* 2001;26:S39–S46

International Standards for Neurologic Classification of Spinal Cord Injury. Chicago: American Spinal Cord Injury Association;2000.

McMichan JC, Michel L, and Westbrook PR. Pulmonary dysfunction following traumatic quadriplegia. *JAMA* 1980;243:528

Panjabi MM, Thibodeau LL, Crisco JJ, et al . What constitutes spinal instability? *Clin Neurosurg* 1988;34:313–339

Pointillart V, Petitjean ME, Wiart L, et al. Pharmacological therapy of spinal cord injury during the acute phase. *Spinal Cord* 2000;38:71–76

Sekhon LHS and Fehlings MG. Epidemiology, demographics, and pathophysiology of acute spinal cord injury. *Spine* 2001;26(24 Suppl): S2–S12

13 Infectious Disorders

Wendy C. Ziai

Definitions, Etiology, and Presentation

♦ Meningitis: Inflammation of the pia and arachnoid membranes (meninges) that surround the brain and spinal cord:
  – Acute: <4 wk duration
  – Recurrent: Multiple acute episodes, each <4 wk
  – Chronic: >4 wk duration
♦ Acute aseptic meningitis:
  – Most common form of meningitis
  – Negative routine screening cultures
  – Starts with high-grade fever and severe headache
  – Associated symptoms: nausea, vomiting, pharyngitis, diarrhea, neck stiffness, photophobia
  – Rapid and complete recovery is the usual course
  – Commonly caused by viral infection
  – 55–70% of cases caused by enteroviruses (echovirus, coxsackie A and B, poliovirus, enteroviruses)
  – Other important causes:
    • Human immunodeficiency virus (HIV) at primary infection and at seroconversion
    • Parasites: Rickettsiae and Mycoplasma
    • Noninfectious disorders: Autoimmune diseases, malignancies, drug reactions (sulfa drugs, nonsteroidal anti-inflammatory drugs [NSAIDs] [e.g., Ibuprofen, isoniazid])
♦ Acute septic meningitis:
  – Bacterial infection of the meninges
  – Neurologic emergency
  – Mortality up to 25%; morbidity up to 60%

From: *Current Clinical Neurology: Handbook of Neurocritical Care*
Edited by: A. Bhardwaj, M. A. Mirski, and J. A. Ulatowski © Humana Press Inc., Totowa, NJ

- Mortality highest in patients with decreased level of consciousness and inadequate antibiotic therapy, and Gram-negative meningitis
- Classic presentation: Fever, headache, reduced alertness, meningeal irritation (Kernig's sign and Brudzinski's sign present in only 50% of children and fewer adults)
- Absence of febrile response may occur in elderly, immunocompromised, inadequate antibiotic treatment
- Seizures occur in 10% of adults and may indicate intracranial mass or cerebral venous sinus thrombosis with hemorrhagic infarction
- Coma can occur in fulminant bacterial meningitis with diffuse cerebral edema, leading to cerebral herniation
- Focal neurologic signs or papilledema develop at some time in 10 to 20% of patients
- Gram-negative meningitis associated with brain swelling in 14% of patients and hydrocephalus in 12%
- Multiple cerebral infarcts may occur secondary to vasculitis
- Specific features by organism:
  • Meningococcal meningitis: petechial or purpural rash, subconjunctival hemorrhages
  • *Haemophilus influenzae*: ataxia and labrynthitis
  • Tuberculous meningitis: cough, fever, night sweats, cranial nerve deficits
  • *Listeria:* rhombencephalitis; cerebrospinal fluid (CSF) profile may appear benign. Magnetic resonance imaging (MRI) is more sensitive
- Systemic manifestations in 22%:
  • Septic shock: 12%
  • Pneumonia: 8%
  • Disseminated intravascular coagulation: 8%
♦ Epidemiology:
- Incidence of *H. Influenzae* meningitis reduced by 94% from 1986 to 1995 as a result of widespread use of conjugated *H. Influenzae* type b vaccine
- Primarily affects children. Therefore median age of bacterial meningitis rose from 15 mo in 1986 to 25 yr in 1995
- Distribution of causative agents of bacterial meningitis in the United States:
  • *Streptococcus pneumoniae*: 47%
  • *Neisseria meningitides*: 25%

- Group B Streptococcus: 13%
- *Listeria monocytogenes*: 8%
- *H. influenzae*: 7%
- Different strains of *H. Influenzae* cause meningitis in adults. Therefore, less decline in incidence rates in adults
- Up to 50% of adult cases infected by nonencapsulated strains of *H. Influenzae*
- Increasing incidence of meningitis associated with Gram-negative nosocomial infections (11% in the1960s; 24% in the1980s)
- Partly attributed to increase in neurosurgical procedures and in immune compromised patients
- High level of penicillin resistance in *Streptococcus pneumoniae* isolates resulting from changes in high-molecular-weight penicillin binding proteins
- Greater than 90% of penicillin resistant isolates remain sensitive to third-generation cephalosporins
- Alcoholics—prone to infection with *L. monocytogenes* and *H. Influenzae*
- Diabetics—prone to infection with Enterobacteriacceae and *Staphylococcus aureus*
- Immunocompromised patients in ICU susceptible to *L. monocytogenes* and *Nocardia asteroides*
- Meningitis after basal skull fracture primarily caused by *Streptococcus pneumoniae*, but increasing trend to Gram-negative organisms; antibiotic prophylaxis not recommended because of possible selection of resistant organisms
- Meningitis after spinal anesthesia—frequently associated with *Pseudomonas aeruginosa*
♦ Recurrent meningitis:
- Infectious and noninfectious causes
- Viruses most likely infectious agents
- Clinical presentation resembles aseptic meningitis
- Mollaret's meningitis: type of recurrent aseptic meningitis associated with Epstein–Barr virus and herpes simplex I virus
♦ Chronic meningitis:
- Nonspecific presentation: variable fever, headache, stiff neck, signs of parenchymal involvement such as altered mental status, seizures, or focal neurologic deficits
- Infectious causes include central nervous system (CNS) tuberculosis and cryptococcus
- Noninfectious causes include neoplasms, neurosarcoidosis, and CNS vasculitis

♦ Tuberculous meningitis:
  – Increasing incidence. Seen in 0.5% of all cases of tuberculosis (TB)
  – Up to 18% of HIV+ patients in endemic areas may have CNS TB
  – Intracranial tuberculomas develop in 10 to 20% of cases of tuberculous meningitis
  – *M. tuberculosis* seeds CNS hematogenously. Forms subpial tuberculomas in brain and spinal cord. Seeds CSF causing meningitis and can cause vascular occlusion as a result of mononuclear infiltration of vessel walls

♦ Fungal meningitis:
  – Generalized meningitis or focal lesions. Basilar meninges typically affected
  – Focal lesions include abscesses, granulomas, vasculitic lesions, and mycotic aneurysms
  – *Cryptococcus*, *Coccidiodes*, *Candida* most frequently present with meningitis. *Aspergillus* usually presents with abscesses
  – Immunocompromised hosts: more indolent chronic course. In nonimmunocompromised may present like other CNS infection
  – Most common complication is hydrocephalus. Shunting frequently required

♦ Encephalitis: Acute infection of brain parenchyma:
  – Prodrome often occurs with fever, headache, myalgia, mild respiratory infection
  – Changes in level of consciousness or personality change may follow
  – Seizures not uncommon. Focal motor seizures affecting face and upper extremities common in Herpes simplex encephalitis (HSE) as a result of frontal and temporal lobe involvement
  – Focal neurologic signs like hemiparesis and aphasia also more common with HSE than other encephalitides
  – Most commonly caused by viral infection: usually affect cerebral hemispheres, but may selectively involve brainstem
  – Direct cellular damage considered less clinically important than delayed hypersensitivity
  – Common causes include arboviruses, exanthem viruses, and mumps although many of undetermined etiology
  – Herpes simplex virus (HSV): up to 15% of cases
  – HSE associated with mortality: 50–70% with significant long-term morbidity in survivors. Seizures, cognitive and behavioral disorders

- Other common viruses include: enteroviruses, lymphocytic choriomeningitis (LCM), togaviruses
- Specific presentations:
  - Parotitis (mumps)
  - Herpetic rash (HSE)
  - Zoster ophthalmicus or Ramsay–Hunt syndrome. Multiple cranial nerve palsies: varicella zoster
  - Diplopia, dysarthria, ataxia (immunocompromised with brainstem HSE)
♦ Brain Abscess: purulent infection of brain parenchyma:
- Most common in children aged 4–7 yr, and in third decade in adults
- Often presents with site-specific focal neurologic deficits, like aphasia and weakness
- Many patients present with signs of increased intracranial pressure (ICP): headache, change in mental status, nausea and vomiting
- Fever less common
- Neck rigidity present in 25% of cases and may indicate associated meningitis
- Seizures, often generalized tonic clonic, occur in up to 40% of cases
- Route of transmission usually contiguous spread from local primary focus: paranasal sinusitis, otitis media, mastoiditis, penetrating head trauma (10%)
- 20% of cases spread hematogenously: usually pulmonary source such as bronchiectasis or lung abscess, or cardiac, from heart valves (infective endocarditis), or conditions causing a right to left shunt. May also come from mouth, skin, gastrointestinal tract
- Single abscess usual with contiguous spread
- Multiple abscesses seen in 20% of cases with hematogenous seeding
- Blood cultures usually negative
- Abscess is polymicrobial in 30–60%
- Anaerobes identified in 30% of isolates
- Most common infectious agents: Streptococcal species (in 40% of brain abscesses), especially *Streptococcus milleri*
- Other organisms include: *Bacteroides* species (in 30%), the *Enterobacteriaceae* family, and *S. aureus*
- Immunosuppressed: consider *L. monocytogenes*, mycobacteria, fungi, parasites
- *S. pyogenes* common in penetrating skull injuries

– Complications from abscess include: strokes caused by cortical thrombophlebitis, rupture of abscess into ventricle or subarachnoid space causing meningitis or ventriculitis and increased intracranial pressure

– Overall mortality from brain abscess approximately 10%

♦ Intracranial extra-axial pyogenic infections: Epidural abscess and subdural empyema are bacterial infections within the extracerebral space:

– Epidural abscess:
  • Usually frontal
  • Present with headache, fever, nausea
  • Rarely neurologic symptoms or complications because of protective effect of adherent dura to overlying skull

– Subdural empyema:
  • Usually over cerebral convexity
  • Presents with altered level of consciousness, focal neurologic deficits, seizures
  • May cause inflammation of brain parenchyma with edema, elevated ICP, septic thrombophlebitis, venous infarction, mass effect

– Either infection may result from trauma, neurosurgical procedure, meningitis, sinusitis, other extracranial source of infection

– Valveless emissary veins allow superfisicial infections to drain into dural sinuses causing thrombophlebitis

– Common organisms include: staphylococci, streptococci, anaerobes (*propionebacterium* and *peptostreptococcus*)

– 40% of cases are polymicrobial

♦ Ventriculitis: pyogenic infection of the ventricular cavity. Criteria for diagnosis: CSF leukocyte count >200/mm^3, or positive culture of ventricular fluid:

– Most common organisms: Staphylococcal species

– 30% of meningitis associated with ventriculitis (90% of neonatal meningitis)

– Consider in patients with meningitis who do not respond quickly to antibiotics

– Often associated with CSF shunts

CNS Infections: Acute Management

♦ Goals:
– Stabilize patient
– Confirm diagnosis of CNS infection
– Start therapy

♦ Stabilize patient:
  – Airway, breathing, circulation
  – Consider possible ICP elevation
  – Evaluate hemodynamic stability—sepsis common
  – Address systemic arterial pressure and cerebral perfusion
  pressure
♦ Diagnosis and early therapy:
  – Obtain CSF access as soon as safe (Table 1)
  – Head computerized tomography (CT) recommended to assess
  risk for cerebral herniation *prior* to CSF access if:
    • Significant alteration in mentation or comatose
    • Focal neurologic deficits
    • Seizures
    • Papilledema
    • Sedation or muscle paralysis
  – If any of the above are present obtain blood cultures and start
  empiric antibiotic therapy prior to CT scan and lumbar puncture
  – Neuroimaging should not delay administration of antibiotics.
  Mortality from delaying antibiotic treatment for CT and lumbar
  puncture (LP) is 10 to 20 times the risk of complications associated with lumbar puncture. Delay of antibiotics also reduces
  potential for complete recovery.
  – Diagnostic sensitivity of CSF not diminished by delaying
  antibiotic therapy by 1 or 2 h after initiating antibiotic therapy as
  long as CSF evaluation includes bacterial antigen testing and
  blood cultures are drawn
  – CSF counterimmunoelectrophoresis, CSF latex agglutination,
  and coagulation tests can detect common bacterial antigens in
  70–100% of patients
  – Perform systemic search to determine non-CNS sources of
  infection (blood, urine, sputum)

Neuroimaging in CNS Infections

♦ Bacterial meningitis:
  – CT usually normal. Subtle findings include: distention of subarachnoid space, followed by enhancement of meninges. MRI
  better modality to detect enhancement of meninges with gadolinium, or infarcts secondary to vasculitis
  – Exceptional findings: subdural effusions (*H. Influenzae* meningitis), brainstem encephalitis (*Listeria*), global cerebral edema,
  cortical infarcts secondary to vasculitis, mild obstructive hydrocephalus, abscess formation

Table 1
Evaluation of CSF

CNS infection	CSF opening pressure	Protein	Glucose	White blood count (WBC)/type	Gram stain/ culture	Other tests	Blood cultures
Bacterial Meningitis	Elevated	Remains elevated for at least 10 d (most resistant to rapid change) >100 mg/dL	Decreased (<50% of serum)	Polymorphonuclear pleocytosis with leukocytes >100/mm^3 in 90%; >1000/ mm^3 in 60%	positive in 60–90%; cultures positive in 80%; reduced rates if partially treated	Increased CSF lactate Latex agglutination tests positive in 50–100%; Bacterial DNA detection + ve in Lyme disease—70–80%; Tuberculosis acid fast stain positive in 35—80%; Touch prep of skin— meningococcal meningitis- positive gm stain in 70%	positive in 50% of cases
Fungal meningitis	Normal to mild elevation	Increased	Low	Modest leukocytosis; usually lymphocytic or monocytic predominance		India ink smears positive in 50–75% of C. Neoformans (but must confirm by culture) ; Latex agglutination for C. Neoformans; complement fixing antibody (CFA) test for IgG antibody in CSF	

Tuberculous meningitis	Usually increased	Increased average 2.6 g/L	Low	Initially may have PMN pleocytosis; usually >500/mm^3; then lymphocyte predominance	Acid-fast bacillus smear positive in 35% at first LP; 80% with three LPs; CSF cultures positive in 3–6 mo in 35% of cases	CT scan shows basilar meningeal enhancement in up to 50%; intraparenchymal tuberculomas show characteristic T2 shortening on MRI
CNS viral infection	Normal to mild elevation	Increased	normal	Lymphocytosis: 50–2000/mm^3	Cultures may be useful; viral culture from brain tissue takes 48 h	PCR (HSE) 98% sensitivity; 94% specificity; 1/3 of cases remain positive long after starting acyclovir; CMV– PCR: 95% specific; 79% sensitive; Toxoplasma 100% specific; 42% sensitive; Arbovirus–IgM antibody detection by ELISA diagnostic
Subdural empyema/ epidural abscess polymorphonuclear	Normal to mild elevation	Increased	normal	10–500/mm^3	Often negative	Serologic testing of acute and convalescent sera may be useful

  - TB meningitis: abnormal CT in 50% with hydrocephalus, superfiscial meningial enhancement in basilar subarachnoid space, cerebral infarcts
  - Ventriculitis: loss of distinct ependymal margin, irregularity of ventricular wall, increased density of ventricular fluid, periventricular edema, hydrocephalus
♦ Encephalitis:
  - MRI flair sequences can be definitive: typical asymmetrical changes in the anterior and medial temporal lobe, inferior frontal lobe, insular cortex, splenium of corpus callosum
  - CT only abnormal after several days: hypodensity and swelling in temporal and insular regions, that may become hemorrhagic
  - Single Photon Emission Computed Tomography (SPECT) may indicate inflammation and neuronal injury in the temporal and frontal lobes, but half of scans are normal in acute stage
♦ Brain abscess:
  - Early cerebritis: poorly marginated subcortical hypodense area on CT
  - Late cerebritis: irregular enhancing rim surrounding a central low-density area
  - Early capsule stage: strongly enhancing collagenous capsule associated with moderate vasogenic edema
  - Late capsule stage: central necrosis
  - Compared to neoplastic lesions, the enhancing rim of the capsule is typically less well developed on the ventricular side of an abscess because of relative differences in vascular supply

Other Diagnostic Tests

♦ Electroencephalogram (EEG): Encephalitis: look for spike and slow wave activity, δ-waves, or triphasic waves that evolve into typical periodic (2–3 Hz) sharp wave complexes (unilateral or bilateral) in temporal regions = periodic lateralized epileptiform discharges (PLEDs). Seen in 84% of typical HSE
♦ Brain biopsy: rarely indicated for diagnosis of HSV encephalitis. Recommended indications for brain biopsy: presence of atypical CSF findings, negative polymerase chain reaction (PCR) and antibody studies, nonspecific magnetic resonance (MR) scan and EEG, or a progressive clinical course despite acyclovir therapy

Management of ICP Elevation

♦ ICP monitor: consider placement based on patient's risk of further neurologic injury and deterioration; no clear guidelines; recommend guidelines adapted from brain trauma literature (*see* Chapter 6): GCS 3–8 with abnormal head CT scan, or a comatose patient with a normal head CT and two or more of the following: Age >40 yr, unilateral or bilateral motor posturing, systolic blood pressure (SBP) <90 mm Hg

Therapeutics

♦ Bacterial meningitis: empiric antibiotic therapy should consider patient age, immune system competence, associated morbidities (*see* Table 2)
  – Immune-competent:
    • Third generation cephalosporin: Ceftriaxone: 2 g q 12h or
    • Cefotaxime: 2 g q 4h plus
    • Vancomycin: 1 g q12h plus
    • Ampicillin: 12 g/d if >50 yr old (more susceptible to *Streptococcus agalactiae* and *L. monocytogenes*)
  – Immunocompromised:
    • Ampicillin: 12 g/d
    • Ceftazidime: 6 g/d
  – Neurosurgical patients:
    • Vancomycin
    • Third generation cephalosporin
  – Steroids: use of steroids in adult central nervous system (CNS) infections is not fully established
  – Decadron may decrease CNS penetration of cephalosporins and vancomycin
  – Prospective randomized trial showed benefits in adults with acute bacterial meningitis. Reduction in risk of unfavorable outcome and mortality. Most evident in patients with pneumococcal meningitis; beneficial effect was not observed for neurologic sequelae, including hearing loss
  – In children with *H. Influenzae* meningitis, steroids decrease rate of sensorineuroal hearing loss and other neurologic sequelae
  – Suggested adult dose of decadron: 4 mg IV q6h for 4 d

Table 2
Antimicrobial Therapy for CNS Infections

Organism	Recommended antimicrobial agent(s)/(daily dose)	Duration of therapy (d)
Bacterial meningitis:		
S. pneumoniae (penicillin resistant)	Cefotaxime (2 g q4-6h) or ceftriaxone (1-2 g q24h) plus vancomycin (1 g q12h)	10–14
N. meningitidis	Penicillin G (4 million units q 4h) or ampicillin (2 g q4h)	7
H. Influenzae type b (β-lactamase positive)	Cefotaxime or ceftriaxone	7
Gram-negative bacilli (not including *Pseudomonas aeruginosa*)	Cefotaxime or ceftriaxone	21
Enterobacteriaceae	Cefotaxime or ceftriaxone	21
P. aeruginosa	Ceftazidime (2 g q8h) plus gentamycin (5 mg/kg divided q 8h)	21
Listeria monocytogenes	Ampicillin (2 g q4h)	14–21
S. aureus (methicillin-sensitive)	Oxacillin (2 g q4h)	10–14
S. aureus (methicillin-resistant)	Vancomycin (1 g q12h)	10–14
Encephalitis:		
Herpes simplex virus	Acyclovir (10 mg/kg q 8h)	10
Cytomegalovirus (CMV),	Gancyclovir (10 mg/kg q12h),	14
Varicella-zoster virus (VZV)	plus foscarnet (180 mg/kg q8h) if on maintenance gancyclovir	
Brain abscess:		
Empiric coverage	Cefotaxime (2 g q4-6h) plus metronidazole (500 mg q8h)	4–8 wk IV plus PO up to 3 mo
Penetrating head trauma	Oxacillin (2g q4h) or vancomycin (1g q12h) plus cefotaxime	
Recent neurosurgery	Vancomycin plus ceftazidime	
Subdural empyema and epidural abscess:		
Empiric	Cefotaxime (2 g q4-6h) plus metronidazole (500 mg q8h); or Piperacillin/tazobactam (3.375 g q6h)	2–6 wk IV

Adapted from **Roos K, Tunkel A.** (1997) Acute bacterial meningitis in children and adults, in: *Infections of the Central Nervous System,* 2nd ed. (Scheld WM, Durack DT, eds.), Philadelphia: Lippincott-Raven, pp. 335–402; and from **Wijdicks EFM.** (2000) Acute bacterial infec-tions of the central nervous system, in: *Neurologic Catastrophes in the Emergency Department,* Boston: Butterworth-Heineman, pp. 183–194.

194

◆ CNS tuberculosis: combination of first four agents (streptomycin can be substituted for Rifampin if not tolerated. Duration of therapy should be at least 6 mo or longer (depending on sensitivities and clinical response). For patients in coma, or with intracranial tuberculomas, decadron is recommended:
  – Isoniazid: 5 mg/kg PO/IM qd
  – Rifampin: 10 mg/kg PO/IV qd
  – Pyrazinamide: 15–30 mg/kg PO qd
  – Ethambutol: 15–25 mg/kg PO qd
  – Streptomycin: 15 mg/kg IM qd
◆ Fungal meningitis: for *Cryptococcus*, *Coccidiodes*, *Candida*, and *Aspergillus*:
  – Amphotericin B: 0.4–0.6 mg/kg/d IV (1.0–1.5 mg/kg/d for *Aspergillus*)
  – Intravenous Amphotericin B combined with flucytosine (37.5 mg/kg q6h) found to reduce relapse rate and clear CSF more rapidly than IV amphotericin alone
  – Intrathecal Amphotericin 0.5 mg three times a week (total dose 20–25 mg) recommended for meningeal coccidiomycosis
  – Monitor hematologic and renal profiles while on therapy
  – HIV+ patients require chronic suppressive therapy:
  – Fluconazole (200 mg/d): Preferred antifungal for prevention of relapses of cryptococcal meningitis
◆ Viral encephalitis:
  – Acyclovir (10 mg/kg every 8 h) IV for 10 d. If relapse, recommend longer course of acyclovir (14 to 21 d)
  – Caution: 10% have reversible elevation in serum creatinine
  – Anticonvulsant therapy if seizures occur
  – Prophylactic anticonvulsants have no proven value
  – Potential benefit of decompressive craniectomy for patients with cerebral edema and impending cerebral herniation: 5/6 patients recovered almost completely with only mild or no neurologic deficits on long-term follow-up
  – For CMV and VZV: Treat with gancyclovir (10 mg/kg bid) for 14 d; add foscarnet (180 mg/kg) every 8 h for patients previously on maintenance-dose gancyclovir
◆ Intracranial extra-axial pyogenic infections:
  – Subdural empyema:
    • Third generation cephalosporin + metronidazole
    • Or piperacillin + tazobactam
  – Early surgical evacuation

- Craniotomy preferred to multiple burr holes
- Continue antibiotics for 2–6 wk
- Antibiotics may be only therapy for fluid collections <1 cm diameter and with rapid clinical improvement

♦ Brain abscess:
- Antibiotic therapy and surgical intervention generally required: drainage by aspiration through burr hole (± stereotactic guidance) or craniotomy
- Empiric antibiotics: Third generation cephalosporin + metronidazole
- If staphylococcal, or history of trauma or recent surgery, add oxacillin or vancomycin
- Treat *P. aeruginosa* with ceftazidime
- Intravenous antibiotics for 4–8 wk, followed by oral antibiotics for up to 3 mo
- Steroid therapy recommended if cerebral edema is significant, especially with early signs of herniation
- Routine steroid therapy controversial because of: potential decreased antibiotic penetration into CNS, decreased collagen formation and glial response and loss of CT scan appearance of ring enhancement with resolving inflammation
- Experimental models suggest decadron may decrease mortality. Human studies have been too small to predict effect on mortality
- Surgical debridement and excision recommended for posterior fossa abscesses
- Aspiration safer if thick fibrotic capsule and impending rupture into ventricles, although repeat operations may be required
- Medical therapy alone reasonable for poor surgical risk patients, multiple small abscesses, high suspicion for Toxoplasma, only cerebritis on CT
- Complications of cerebral abscess: satellite abscesses, ventriculitis, choroid plexitis, purulent meningitis

♦ Ventriculitis:
- Gram-positive: vancomycin (although CNS penetration may be negligible if meningeal inflammatory response is less extensive as a result of prior treatment
- In this case consider intrathecal instillation of antibiotic which may achieve adequate concentrations and be necessary for successful eradication
- *Note*: conventional doses administered into the lumbar sac do not give reliable brain CSF concentrations

- Risks include: hemorrhage, CSF leak, infection, seizures, direct toxicity
- Recommended to obtain CSF levels
- Remove or externalize infected intraventricular device
- Experience with intraventricular administration of antibiotics limited: one report of 50 episodes of shunt related ventriculitis–overall cure rate of only 60%, but systemic antibiotics not used in all patients
- Suggested regimen: vancomycin: 10–20 mg/d with adjustment based on CSF vancomycin concentration for 3–4 d after culture results negative
- Recommended trough concentrations: 10–20 ug/mL
- For Gram-negative ventriculitis, less encouraging results
- Most studies show no significant clinical benefit with intrathecal gentamycin or amikacin
- Reported adverse events: vestibular and auditory dysfunction, clinical encephalopathy, CSF eosinophilia, local tissue irritation

Key Points

♦ CSF analysisis important in making diagnosis and guiding therapy
♦ In suspected acute bacterial meningitis, start antimicrobial treatment prior to CT, preferably after drawing blood cultures
♦ Consider steroids with first dose of intravenous antibiotics and for 4 d
♦ Be aware of systemic and neurologic complications of CNS infection
♦ Reassess patient condition frequently and investigate any change in neurologic condition suggesting occurrence of edema and/or hydrocephalus

Suggested Reading

Bell BA and Britton JA. Brain Abscess, in: *Infections of the Central Nervous System.* (Lambert HP, ed.), Philadelphia: Decker; 1991: 361–373.

Berenguer J, Moreno S, Laguna F, et al. Tuberculous meningitis in patients infected with the human immunodeficiency virus. *N Engl J Med* 1992;326:668.

De Gans J, Van de Beek, D., et al. Dexamethasone in adults with bacterial meningitis. *NEJM* 2002;347:1549–1456.

Coyle P. Overview of acute and chronic meningitis, in: *Neurologic Clinics: Central Nervous System Infections,* vol. 17. Philadelphia: WB Saunders; 1999:691–710.

Kita M, Laskowitz DT, and Kolson DL. Central nervous system infections, in: _Critical Care Neurology._ (Miller DH and Raps EC, eds.), Boston: Butterworth-Heinemann; 1999:279–330.

Roos K and Tunkel A. Acute bacterial meningitis in children and adults, in:_,Infections of the Central Nervous System_, ,vol. 2. (Scheld WM and Durack DT, eds.), Philadelphia: Lippincott-Raven Publishers; 1997: 335–402.

Seydoux C. and Francioli P. Bacterial brain abscesses: factors influencing mortality and sequelae. _Clin Infect Dis_ 1992;15:394.

Talan DA, Hoffman JR, Yoshikawa TT, Overturf GD. Role of empiric parenteral antibiotics prior to lumbar puncture in suspected bacterial meningitis: state of the art. _Rev Infect Dis_ 1988;10:365–376

Whitley RJ, Soong SJ, Linneman C. Jr., et al. NIAID Collaborative Antiviral Study Group. Herpes simplex encephalitis: clinical assessment. _JAMA_ 1982;247:317.

Wijdicks EFM. Neurologic manifestations of bacterial infection and sepsis, in: _Neurologic Complications of Critical Illness_, 2nd ed. New York: Oxford University Press; 2002:93–122.

14   Neuromuscular Disorders

Michel T. Torbey

Nerve and Muscle Disorders Commonly Admitted to the Intensive Care Unit (ICU)

♦ Guillain–Barre Syndrome
♦ Myasthenia Gravis
♦ Tetanus
♦ Botulism
♦ Organophosphate toxicity

Common Reasons for ICU Admission

♦ Ventilatory failure (most common)
♦ Pneumonia
♦ Deep venous thrombosis (DVT) and/or pulmonary embolus
♦ Autonomic dysfunction
♦ Cardiac arrythmias

General Clinical Manifestations of Respiratory Failure

♦ Increased respiratory rate and use of accessory muscles
♦ Weak shoulder shrug and head elevation
♦ Absence of paradoxic inward movement of the abdominal wall muscles with inspiration
♦ Complaints of air hunger
♦ Inability to count to 20 on one breath

Guillain–Barre Syndrome

♦ Major cause of acute flaccid paralysis in healthy individuals
♦ Worldwide incidence of Guillain–Barre syndrome (GBS) varies between 0.6 and 1.9 cases per 100,000 per year

From: *Current Clinical Neurology: Handbook of Neurocritical Care*
Edited by: A. Bhardwaj, M. A. Mirski, and J. A. Ulatowski © Humana Press Inc., Totowa, NJ

♦ Two age peaks with minor peak in young adults and a second larger one in the fifth through eighth decades of life
♦ The occurrence rate is slightly higher for men than for women, and higher for whites than for blacks
♦ Preceding illnesses such as flu-like symptoms or a diarrheal illness may occur 1–3 wk before onset of symptoms in two thirds of patients.
♦ Diagnosis based on progressive areflexic weakness of more than one limb
♦ Most common preceding infections include Campylobacter jejuni, cytomegalovirus (CMV), and Epstein–Barr virus (EBV)

Clinical Spectrum

♦ Acute inflammatory demyelinating polyneuropathy (AIDP):
  – Most prevalent form
  – Accounts for 85–90% of cases
♦ Acute motor axonal neuropathy (AMAN):
  – Less severe axonal form
  – Described in children and young adults in northern China
♦ Acute motor sensory axonal neuropathy (AMSAN):
  – More severe form of GBS,
  – Patients present with a fulminant onset of paralysis following a prodromal illness
♦ Miller–Fisher syndrome (MFS):
  – Characterized by ophthalmoplegia, ataxia, and areflexia
  – Associated with antibodies to GQ1b ganglioside

Recommendations for Admission to the Neurologic Critical Care Unit

♦ Rapid progression of motor weakness including respiratory muscles
♦ Presence of bulbar dysfunction and bilateral facial palsy
♦ Autonomic dysfunction
♦ Arrhythmia and bradycardia
♦ Medical complications:
  – Deep vein thrombosis, pulmonary embolus
  – Myocardial infarction
  – Sepsis

Patterns of Respiratory Function in GBS

♦ Gradual decline: <30% reduction in vital capacity (VC) > 24 h
♦ Rapid decline: >30% reduction in VC in <24 h
♦ No decline: 86% will not require ventilation

Predictors of Mechanical Ventilation

♦ Clinical predictors:
  – Presence of bulbar dysfunction and bilateral facial palsy
  – Autonomic dysfunction
  – Shorter time to peak disability following the onset of symptoms
♦ Radiological predictors:
  – Pulmonary infiltrates
  – Atelectasis
  – Pleural effusion

Recommendations for Intubation and Weaning in GBS Patients

♦ Indications for intubation:
  – Clinical evidence of fatigue or severe oropharyngeal weakness
  – Respiratory function:
    • Vital capacity 15–20 mL/kg or <1 L
    • Maximal inspiratory pressure <30 cm H_2O
    • Maximal expiratory pressure <40 cm H_2O
    • Reduction > 30% of baseline VC
    • PO_2 < 70 mm Hg on room air
♦ Indications for weaning:
  – Forced vital capacity (FVC) >10 mL/kg
  – Negative inspiratory force (NIF) > 20 cm of H_2O
  – Satisfactory oxygenatory and ventilatory functions.
  – Extubation with direct laryngoscopic or fiberoptic visualization or after a cuff test in cases of prolonged intubation

Autonomic Dysfunction and GBS

♦ Important cause of death in severe GBS
♦ Risk of dysautonomia is high in patients with tetraplegia, respiratory failure, or bulbar involvement
♦ Frequent manifestations are sinus tachycardia or bradycardia, hypertension, and labile blood pressure (BP)
♦ In severe cases of dysautonomia placement of a temporary pacemaker may be needed
♦ Hypotension is best managed with fluid administration:
  – If hypotension is refractory to volume repletion, treatment with an α agonist such as phenylephrine, a short acting vasopressor, may be indicated. Consider addition of midodrine
  – Hypertension may follow a hypotensive episode or may occur independently

– Generally, no treatment is necessary unless there is evidence of end-organ injury or unless the mean arterial pressure (MAP) exceeds 120 mmHg

Nutrition in GBS

♦ Enteral feeding is started as soon as possible
♦ Initial replacement at 30 to 40 kcal/kg nonprotein calories and 2.0–2.5 g protein/Kg
♦ Weekly 24 h urine samples are obtained to calculate nitrogen balance and estimate protein needs
♦ Initiate formulas at full strength unless there is delayed gastric emptying or the patient presents with severe protein-caloric malnutrition

Pain Control

♦ Frequent repositioning may be helpful initially
♦ Nonsteroidal anti-inflammatory drugs are often effective:
– Ketorolac im injection of 30 mg and than 15 mg to 30 mg IM every 6 h
♦ Narcotics may be needed to provide appropriate patient comfort
♦ Nortriptyline may be an effective alternative:
– Should be avoided in patients with autonomic dysfunction
♦ Valproic acid, carbamezepine, and gabapentin may be used with neuropathic pain

Treatment of GBS

Figure 1 describes the Algorithm for Treatment of GBS

Management Pearls for GBS

♦ Ventilatory failure does not correlate well with the general neuromuscular examination
♦ Current ICU practice is trending toward earlier intubation
♦ Blood-gas analysis is not particularly useful to decide whether patient needs intubation
♦ Hypoxia is usually a late occurrence. Hypercarbia eventually leads to decreased mental status resulting in hypoventilation and hypoxemia

Myasthenia Gravis

Epidemiology

♦ Autoimmune disorder caused by antibodies against acetylcholine receptors (ACHR) of the postsynaptic portion of the neuromuscular junction (NMJ)

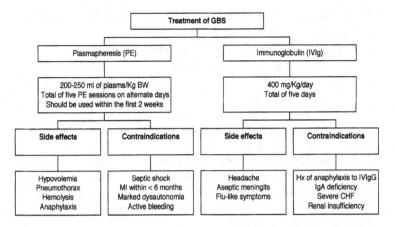

Fig. 1. Algorithm for the treatment of GBS

- Prevalence rate of 0.5–14.2 per 100,000
- May occur at any age
- Women more frequently affected than men (3:2) and acquire the disease at a younger age. Men tend to develop the disease later in life

Clinical Features

- Cardinal features are weakness and fatiguabiliy
- Weakness has predilection for ocular muscles
- 70% of patients present with ptosis or extraocular muscle weakness

Commonly Used Anticholinesterase Drugs in Myasthenia Gravis

- Neostigimine Bromide (Prostigimine)
- Neostigimine methyl sulfate (Prostigimine)
- Pyridostigmine Bromide (Mestinon): 15 mg PO q2–3h
- 0.5 mg IM, IV q2–3h
- 60 mg PO q3–4h
- 2 mg IM, IV q3–4h
- Parenteral dose is 1/30 the oral dose

Diagnosis

- Tensilon Test (edrophonium):
  - Short-acting inhibitor of acetylcholinesterase.
  - For best result a placebo control should be used

- Atropine is sometimes necessary to control against muscarinic side effects:
  • Bradycardia, nausea, and increased salivation
- BP and pulse should be monitored
- Tensilon dose:
  • 10 mg in adults
  • 0.2 mg/kg in children
  • 2 mg is infused initially, if no side effect in 30 s, the remaining 8 mg may be given
- It is important to choose an objective clinical sign of weakness to monitor responsiveness to the medication, such as ptosis, ophthalmoparesis, or dysarthria
- Patient should be observed for the duration of action of mestinon usually 2–20 min:
  • Duration may be longer if patient is treated with prednisone (up to 2 h)
♦ Laboratory evidence:
  - Acetylcholine receptor antibodies:
    • Found in 86% of Myasthenia Gravis (MG) patients
    • 71% in ocular MG
    • The severity of myasthenia does not correlate with the concentration of ACHR antibodies
  - Striatal antibody:
    • Found in 80% of patients with MG and thymoma
♦ Electro-diagnostic studies
  - Repetitive nerve stimulation (RNS) at a frequency of 2–3 Hz produces a decremental response greater than 10%
  - If RNS is negative at rest, the muscle is exercised for 1 min followed by RNS at 0 s, 30 s, 1 min, 2 min, and 3 min after exercise
  - A positive decremental response during RNS is seen in 77% of myasthenics
♦ Single fiber EMG:
  - Most sensitive test for myasthenia
  - Abnormalities seen in 92% of patients including those who lack ACHR antibodies or who have normal RNS tests

Pearls in MG

♦ Patients who have pure ocular myasthenia may not have any abnormality in these tests, making diagnosis extremely difficult
♦ Myasthenia does not affect the pupil

♦ A positive Tensilon test is strongly suggestive of MG, but positive tests have also been reported in patients who have intracranial tumors, Lambert–Eaton myasthenic syndrome, botulism, and amyotrophic lateral sclerosis

♦ Tensilon test should not be used in patients with respiratory distress

♦ When there is a doubt about results of Tensilon test in a myasthenic crisis, all anticholinesterase medications should be stopped for 72 h

Crisis in MG

♦ Two type of crisis usually seen:
- Myasthenic crisis
- Cholinergic crisis

Myasthenic Crisis

♦ Approximately 15–20% of myasthenic patients will experience one episode of myasthenic crisis

♦ Myasthenic crisis appears more frequently in patients who have thymoma

♦ Precipitating factors:
- Infection (38%)
- Medication changes, particularly initiation, and withdrawal of corticosteroids
- Aspiration pneumonitis
- Upper airway obstruction
- Pregnancy
- Surgery

♦ For one third of the patients, no precipitating factor can be found.

Cholinergic Crisis

♦ Patients may increase their intake of anticholinergic medications that can lead to weakness

♦ Usually associated with signs of excessive cholinergic activity:
- Miosis
- Diarrhea
- Increased salivation
- Abdominal cramps
- Bradycardia

♦ It is often difficult to differentiate cholinergic crisis from myasthenic crisis:

– A test dose of Tensilon could be used to differentiate myasthenic from cholinergic crisis. Symptoms improve after administration of tensilon in a myasthenic crisis

– It may be difficult to assess a response adequately in an apprehensive patient

Commonly Used Drugs to be Avoided in MG

♦ Quinidine
♦ Procainamide
♦ Propranolol
♦ Thyroid hormone
♦ Phenytoin
♦ Carbamazepine
♦ Morphine
♦ Aminoglycoside
♦ Bactrim
♦ Tetracyclines
♦ Clindamycin
♦ Verapamil
♦ Diltiazem
♦ Diazepam
♦ Morphine

Tetanus

Epidemiology

♦ Incidence is estimated to be between 500,000 and 1 million cases per year worldwide
♦ Male to female ratio of 3:2.
♦ Clostridium tetani, a spore-forming Gram-positive bacillus, is implicated in the pathophysiology of tetanus
♦ Risk factors include:
  – Wounds and lacerations
  – Intravenous drug use
  – Diabetes
  – Lack of immunization

Clinical Features

♦ Trismus or "lockjaw" most common initial symptom (50–75% of cases) Facial muscle contraction (*Risus sardonicus*)
♦ Nuchal rigidity and dysphagia

♦ As the disease spreads, generalized muscle spasms occur, either spontaneously or to minor stimuli
♦ Mental status not affected
♦ Cranial nerve palsies occur uniquely in cephalic tetanus:
  – CN VII is most often involved, followed by the VI, III, IV, and XII in decreasing order of frequency

Diagnosis

♦ No laboratory tests to diagnose or rule out tetanus
♦ Diagnosis made on clinical grounds alone
♦ Spatula test can be helpful
  – 94% sensitivity and 100% specificity
  – Consists of a spatula inserted into the pharynx
  – If patient gags and tries to expel the spatula, test is negative for tetanus
  – If patient bites the spatula because of reflex masseter spasm, the test is positive for tetanus
  – Airway cart should be at the bedside when performing this test

Therapy and Critical Care of Tetanus

♦ Respiratory Failure:
  – Early tracheostomy is preferred to avoid laryngeal spasms precipitated by the presence of an endotracheal tube
♦ Autonomic instability:
  – Occurs several days after the onset of generalized spasms
  – Fatality rate 11–28%.
  – Dysrhythmias and myocardial infarction most common fatal events
  – Labetalol is recommended as a balanced agent for hypertension and tachycardia. Morphine and fentanyl may produce similar control
♦ Muscle spasm:
  – Benzodiazepines are the drug of choice because of their GABA-agonist and sedative properties
  – For severe cases, paralytics may be needed:
    • Vecuronium is an ideal agent for immediate and long-term control because of its minimal cardiovascular effects
    • Succinylcholine should be avoided because of the risk of hyperkalemia

♦ Neutralizing agents:
  − Human tetanus immunoglobulin (HTIG):
    • Neutralize circulating tetanospasmin.
    • Preferred dose is 500 iu given once a day.
  − Metronidazole is the drug of choice to prevent on-going production of toxin
♦ Supportive care:
  − Patients should be placed in a quiet dark environment
  − Because of the recurrence of tetanus in nonimmunized survivors, it is recommended to vaccinate all survivors

Botulism

♦ It is caused by neurotoxin of the bacterium Clostridium botulinum
♦ Nearly all of these new cases have occurred in iv drug users

Clinical Features

♦ Clinical presentations are stereotypical:
  − Signs and symptoms related to oculobulbar muscle weakness
  − Descending pattern of weakness
  − Limb and ocular weakness are usually bilateral but can be asymmetric
  − Sensory system and mentation are usually spared
  − Autonomic signs and symptoms are commonly seen in botulism

Diagnosis

Laboratory Features

♦ Detection of toxin in patient's serum, stool, or wound
♦ If the delay in securing serum samples is >2 d after ingestion of the toxin, the chance of obtaining a positive test is <30%
♦ Only 36% of stool cultures are positive after 3 d

Electrodiagnostic Features

♦ Sensory nerve amplitudes, velocities, and latencies are normal
♦ Motor conduction velocities are normal
♦ Decremental response of the MAP to slow rates of nerve stimulation (2–3 Hz)
♦ Post-tetanic facilitation can be found in some affected muscles
♦ Needle EMG studies reveal an increased number of brief polyphasic motor unit action potentials and spontaneous denervation potentials
♦ Single-fiber EMG studies reveal increased jitter and blocking

Treatment

♦ Mainly supportive
♦ Special attention to respiratory status
♦ Elective intubation should be considered for those at risk for respiratory failure
♦ Most patients will not require a tracheostomy
♦ Autonomic signs and symptoms are commonly seen in botulism
♦ Patients with severe postural hypotension may require midodrine or florinef therapy

Antitoxin Administration

♦ Remains a controversial therapy
♦ Associated 2% risk of allergic reactions
♦ To be of benefit, antitoxin must be given early

Ach Release Promoters

♦ Guanidine and 4-aminopyridine (4-AP) have been reported to improve ocular muscle and limb muscle strength in some patients without any benefit for respiratory paralysis
♦ These two drugs enhance the release of Ach from nerve terminals

Organophosphate Intoxication

♦ Organophosphates irreversibly inhibit cholinesterases including acetylcholinesterases (AchE)
♦ Their potential use in chemical warfare continues to be a serious concern

Clinical Presentation

♦ Symptoms may begin within 3 h of exposure and may progress to death within 10 h
♦ Two types of symptoms: muscarinic and nictonic
♦ Muscarinic symptoms:
  – Reflect the AchE inhibition at autonomic synapses
  – These include miosis, conjunctival hyperemia, rhinorrhea and drooling, bronchospasms with wheezing and coughing, increased bronchial secretion with airway obstruction, respiratory distress, pulmonary edema, laryngeal spasms, sweating, bradycardia, hypotension, loss of bowel and bladder control

♦ Nicotinic effects:
  – Reflect AchE inhibition at the NMJ
  – Fasciculations are first seen in the eyelids, spread to the face
  and calves, and then become generalized. This occurs during the
  first 24 h and is followed by weakness or paralysis, depending on
  the severity of the intoxication
  – Paralysis involves all skeletal muscles, including those of respiration, with labored, shallow, rapid breathing
♦ Severe intoxication ultimately results in confusion, ataxia,
dysarthria, and absent reflexes and may progress to coma, tonic-
clonic seizures
♦ In most patients, complete recovery is expected within 1 to 3 wk
depending on the severity of intoxication and the effectiveness of the
initial therapy

Diagnosis

Laboratory Features

♦ Serum levels of organophosphates and cholinesterase activity
should be obtained
♦ Serum cholinesterase is markedly decreased early in the course
♦ Serum organophosphates levels, initially elevated, decrease rapidly over the first 48 h as they are cleared from the blood to other
body tissues

Electrophysiological Features

♦ Repetitive firing of the single evoked compound muscle action
potential

Therapy and Critical Care of Organophosphate Toxicity

♦ Admission to ICU is recommended for BP, VC, and mental status
monitoring
♦ Endotracheal intubation and mechanical ventilation may be
required
♦ Removing the patients from further exposure is very important:
  – Gastric lavage with water is essential
  – Contamination of skin and mucous membranes requires fre-
  quent washing

♦ Although seizures are rare anticonvulsant therapy is advised
♦ Use atropine to treat muscarinic side effects:
 – 1–2 mg every hour to control excessive pulmonary or bronchial secretion over the first 4–5 d
♦ Pralidoxime, a cholinesterase reactivator, should be used within few hours before phosphorylated AchE becomes resistant to reactivation:
 – If used in severe intoxication, 1 g of pralidoxime is given IV at a rate less than 500 mg/min. If weakness persists after 20 min this dosage may be repeated

Key Points

♦ Neuromuscular syndromes can present with rapid progression involving respiratory failure
♦ Dysautonomia may occur frequently
♦ Treatment in ICU involves support of cardiopulmonary systems and preventing side effects of bed ridden state (DVT, urinary tract infection [UTI], decubiti)
♦ Rehabilitation is needed to pevent contractures and compression neuopathies

Suggested Readings

Bella I and Chad DA. Neuromuscular disorders and acute respiratory failure. *Neuro. Clin* 1998;16(2):391–417.
Cherington M. Botulism. *Semin Neurol* 1990;10(1):27–31.
Drachman DB. Myasthenia gravis. *N Engl J Med* 1994;330(25):1797–1810.
Hund EF, Borel CO, Cornblath DR, Hanley DF, and McKhann GM. Intensive management and treatment of severe Guillain–Barre syndrome. *Crit Care Med* 1993;21(3):433–446.
Lotti M, Becker CE, and Aminoff MJ. Organophosphate polyneuropathy: pathogenesis and prevention. *Neurology* 1984;34(5):658–662.
Oh SJ, Kim DE, Kuruoglu R, Bradley RJ, and Dwyer D. Diagnostic sensitivity of the laboratory tests in myasthenia gravis. *Muscle Nerve* 1992;15(6):720–724.
Plasma Exchange/Sandoglobulin Guillain–Barre Syndrome Trial Group. Randomised trial of plasma exchange, intravenous immunoglobulin, and combined treatments in Guillain–Barre syndrome. *Lancet* 1997;349(9047):225–230.

Ropper A, Wijdicks E, and Truaux B. *Guillain–Barre Syndrome.* Philadelphia: FA Davis; 1991.

The Guillain–Barré syndrome Study Group. Plasmapheresis and acute Guillain–Barré syndrome. *Neurology* 1985;35(8):1096–1104.

Trujillo MH, Castillo A, Espana J, Manzo A, and Zerpa R. Impact of intensive care management on the prognosis of tetanus. Analysis of 641 cases. *Chest* 1987;92(1):63–65

15 Status Epilepticus

Marek A. Mirski

Definition

♦ Status Epilepticus (SE): a seizure persisting for a sufficient length of time or is repeated frequently enough to produce a fixed and enduring epileptic condition:
  – Specific duration of unremitting seizures historically were arbitrarily assigned to 30 min by experts in the field
  – Subsequently shorter seizure epochs have been emphasized as SE
  – Based on typical seizure duration of 1–2 min, SE should likely be considered in seizure events >5–10 min in length
  – Some reports of 10–29 min seizures having spontaneous resolution without therapy, but consensus is that this represents a small population, and a higher risk-benefit ratio exists in not treating such patients as SE

Epidemiology

♦ 100,000–150,000 patients/yr estimated in the United States with mortality 20–25%
♦ Only 0.2% of intensive care unit (ICU) admission diagnoses
♦ Data likely underestimate true incidence of SE especially when all types are considered
♦ Nonconvulsive SE may occur in as many as 8–34% of neurologically ill patients in an ICU setting who are in coma of unclear etiology

Subtypes of SE: Three Major Groupings

♦ Generalized Convulsive SE (GCSE):
  – Classic motor SE

From: *Current Clinical Neurology: Handbook of Neurocritical Care*
Edited by: A. Bhardwaj, M. A. Mirski, and J. A. Ulatowski © Humana Press Inc., Totowa, NJ

- May be overt or have subtle motor manifestations, especially if SE is prolonged
- By far most commonly reported SE type
♦ Focal Motor SE (FMSE) or epilepsy partialis continuans:
- Single limb or side of face most common
♦ Nonconvulsive SE (NCSE):
- Current umbrella term for wide spectrum of continuous nonmotor seizures
- May encompass primary generalized SE, such as absence SE having stereotypic electroencephalogram (EEG), to secondary generalized seizures with variable EEG features.
- Other terms within NCSE: complex-partial SE, subtle SE, nontonic-clonic SE, subclinical SE
- Hallmark is diminishment of neurological exam secondary to the seizure, but patient may present from being awake/ambulatory to coma. The true incidence of this subtype of SE unknown, and likely under recognized
- A recent trend gives label of NCSE to severe anoxic/ischemic encephalopathy, when EEG spikes are present

Anatomy of SE

♦ Partial or focal SE:
- Single focus with local spread
- EEG usually capable of identifying focus, unless deep or medial cortical area (i.e., like deep hippocampus)
♦ Bihemispheric or generalized:
- Commonly focal cortical nidus with rapid spread (may be too rapid for EEG to detect)
- Termed "secondary" generalization.
- Such seizures spread via cortical networks or cortical–subcortical circuits
- "Primary" generalized seizure (e.g., absence) probably utilize brainstem/subcortical structures in mediation and propagation

Etiologies of SE

♦ Causes of seizures may be caused by primary pathology in the patient, or from iatrogenic causes
♦ Regarding etiology of SE on admission to hospital, anticonvulsant noncompliance, alcohol withdrawal, and other drug toxicity are most common precipitants per data obtained during the 1980s as well as more recently (*see* Table 1).

Table 1
Causes of SE at an Urban Public Hospital Over Two Decades

Etiology	*1980s (%)* (n = 157)	*1970s (%)* (n = 98)
AET noncompliance	26	26
ETOH-related	24	15
Drug toxicity	10	10
CNS infection	8	4
Cerebral tumor	6	4
Trauma	5	3
Refractory epilepsy	5	—
Stroke	4	15
Metabolic disorders	4	8
Cardiac arrest	4	4
Unknown	5	15

Adapted from **Lowenstein DH.** 1999.

♦ Seizures in the ICU are particularly prone to be as a consequence of drug toxicity or rapid changes in electrolyte and metabolic condition as depicted (Table 2)

♦ Particular to an ICU setting and critical illness, nonneurological injuries such as metabolic abnormalities, sepsis, and drug toxicity comprise >30–35% of all seizures, of which SE can be complicating sequelae

Morbidity From SE

♦ Generalized convulsive SE (GCSE):

– There is clear evidence of association for systemic complications as well as direct neuronal injury as a consequence of unremitting seizure activity (Table 3)

– Seizures lasting more than one hour represent an independent predictor of poor outcome (mortality odds ration of 10)

– Certain regions of brain are particularly vulnerable to the effects of SE, and these regions typically have high excitatory amino acid–receptor activity

– Most vulnerable brain regions to SE:

• Hippocampal complex

• Pyramidal cells of cerebellum

• Amygdala

Table 2
Common Etiologies of Seizures in the ICU

Neurological Pathology
  Neurovascular
    Stroke
    Arteriovenous malformations
    Hemorrhage
  Tumor
    Primary
    Metastatic
  Central nervous system (CNS) infection
    Abscess
    Meningitis
    Encephalitis
  Inflammatory disease
    Vasculitis
    Acute disseminated encephalomyelitis
  Traumatic head injury
    Contusion
    Hemorrhage
  Primary epilepsy
  Primary CNS metabolic disturbance (inherited)
Complications of critical illness
  Hypoxia/ischemia
  Drug/substance toxicity
    Antibiotics
    Antidepressants
    Antipsychotics
    Bronchodilators
    Local anesthetics
    Immunosuppressives
    Cocaine
    Amphetamines
    Phencyclidine
  Drug/substance withdrawal
    Barbiturates
    Benzodiazepines
    Opioids
    Alcohol
  Infection fever (febrile seizures)
  Metabolic abnormalities
    Hyponatremia
    Hypophosphatemia
    Hypoglycemia
    Renal/hepatic dysfunction
    Surgical injury (craniotomy)

Adapted from **Varelas P and Mirski MA.**, 2001.

Table 3
Associated Complications of GCSE

Systemic
  Acidosis
  Hyperthermia
  Rhabdomyolysis
  Renal failure
  Arrhythmias
  Trauma
  Impaired V/Q matching
  Onemonia
Neurological
  Direct excitotoxic injury
  Epiliptogenic foci
  Synaptic reorganization
  Impaired protein synthesis

Adapted from **Varelas P and Mirski MA.** ,2001.

- Middle cortical lamina
- Thalamus
  - Local, cortical inhibitory circuits that are normally present to assist in limiting seizure duration become ineffective during SE. Seizures themselves augment this disinhibition (early neuronal injury)
  - As a consequence, the longer duration of SE, the more difficult it is to terminate
- Nonconvulsive SE (NCSE):
  - Equally strong consensus exists for not aggressively treating absence SE
  - Apart from the altered cognition during the seizure that may be disabling, there is no evidence that permanent morbidity has been attributed to this form of SE
  - Thus, therapy should be directed toward chronic prevention of the attacks
  - In other subtypes of NCSE, the data are less clear. In the classic form of ambulatory NCSE, again little evidence exists to support permanent injury from SE, although days or weeks of memory disturbance have been reported
  - Appropriate treatment should be instituted, but this condition fails to qualify as a true emergency. In hospitalized patients, certainly in the ICU, the diagnosis of NCSE usually is associated

Table 4
Typical Presentation of GCSE and NCSE SE

Classic GCSE	Generalized spike or sharp wave pattern that begins from a normal background rhythm. SE is characterized by an unremitting spike activity or, more commonly, a crescendo-decrescendo pattern of major motor ictal periods interspersed with lower voltage paroxysmal activity. No abrupt termination or "post-ictal depression" is observed as following simple seizures
NCSE	EEG is variable, with a number of EEG patterns being recognized (*see* "Subtypes of SE"). Generally, seizures such as complex-partial status resemble their non-nonSE counterparts

with moderate to severe cerebral injury as following an anoxic-ischemic event or trauma

– Associating the effects of NCSE on direct neuronal injury is difficult in this setting, although most epileptologists agree that in such scenarios, the presence of continuous paroxysmal activity may accentuate injury incurred by the primary insult

– Therefore, it is prudent to attempt therapy as rapidly as is feasible

Monitoring

♦ EEG is critical in the correct diagnosis of SE, and for monitoring of therapeutic response

♦ Tables 4–5 list common EEG features of GCSE and NCSE

♦ Figure 1 illustrates the onset of GCSE in a patient that is pharmacologically paralyzed. The panel illustrates the EEG onset of a single major convulsive seizure during SE. The bottom panel (B) records the termination of the major motor seizure, with the background not yielding to a flattened pattern, but continuing with paroxysms that will build to yield another major clinical ictal event

♦ Figure 2 represents a case of complex partial SE. The first portion of the record shows predominant left temporal accentuation.

– The second half of the recording (Fig 2) in this 18 yr-old patient demonstrates a rapid 6/s ictal activity that follows the generalized spiking seen in the first half

Table 5
Electroencephalogram Criteria for Nonconvulsive Seizures

Primary	Repetitive generalized or focal spikes, sharp waves, spike-and-wave, or sharp-and-slow complexes at >3/s
	As above but <3/s, but also meeting secondary criteria no. 4 (below)
	Sequential rhythmic waves along with secondary criteria 1,2,3 ±4
Secondary	Incrementing onset: increase in voltage and/or increase/decrease in frequency
	Decrementing offset: decrease in voltage or frequency
	Post-discharge slowing or voltage attenuation
	Significant improvement in clinical state or EEG with anticonvulsant therapy

Adapted from **Brenner RP.**, 2002.

– Although there is yet no consensus on the EEG diagnosis of NCSE (Fig. 3), there have been criteria proposed for a simple nonconvulsive seizure, which may aid in supporting a finding of NCSE
– Some notable associated EEG waveforms are controversial as to whether they represent ictal activity, in particular the periodic lateralizing epileptic discharges (PLEDs if unilateral, BIPLEDs if bilateral/independent, and PEDs if focal or bilateral/uniform) and triphasic waves (TW)
– Figure 3 shows the common combination of both PLEDs and frank electrographic seizure occurring as a continuum
– Many epileptologists regard PLEDs in this context as being an interictal event, whereas others disagree and consider them as continuation of the seizure
– Such a perspective would necessitate treating PLEDs, even if not coincident with recognizable classic EEG ictal periods
– Regardless, the presence of PLEDs suggests severe underlying neuronal injury, with BIPLEDs even worse (mortality of 61% in the latter group compared to 29% in the former)
♦ Obtaining an EEG early when SE is suspected is helpful in establishing the diagnosis of seizure, evaluate for a possible epileptic focus, and to evaluate for residual, nonclinical epileptiform activity:

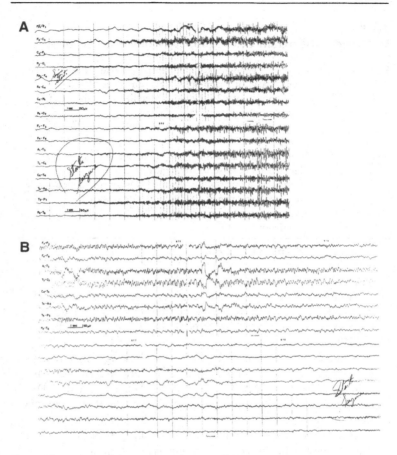

Fig. 1. The onset of GCSE in a pharmacologically paralyzed patient.
Panel B represents subsequent continuation of EEG record in Panel A.
Reproduced from **Niedermeyer E.**, 1993:534 with permission.

– This is true even for convulsive seizures that are treated rapidly
and the patient returns to their baseline level of wakefulness and
cognition
– It is not uncommon for patients to present to the Emergency
Department with motor manifestations convincing of SE, only to
be proven as pseudo-seizures once EEG monitoring is enabled
– Similarly, residual epileptiform activity may be evidence for
NCSE

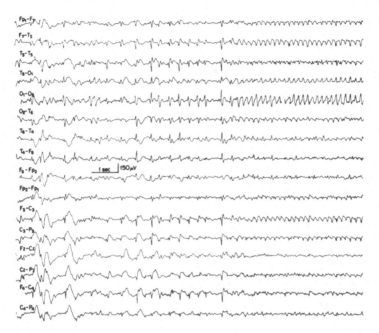

Fig. 2. Patient with complex partial status epilepticus (CPSE).
Reproduced from **Niedermeyer E.**, 1993:537 with permission.

♦ For ongoing SE, EEG (preferably continuous) is mandatory to
ensure effective treatment:
  – Commonly, convulsive SE is incompletely treated with residual
  subtle CSE or NCSE despite cessation of motor ictal activity
  – Some clinical reports suggest residual electrographic seizures
  in almost 50% of patients with GCSE, and a 10–20% incidence of
  NCSE in those patients treated for GCSE with cessation of motor
  seizure activity

Treatment

♦ For the most common SE–GCSE, a variety of algorithms and
agents have been used during the past 20 yr, and new drugs are being
continuously investigated
♦ Nevertheless, some standards for therapy appear well supported by
clinical data

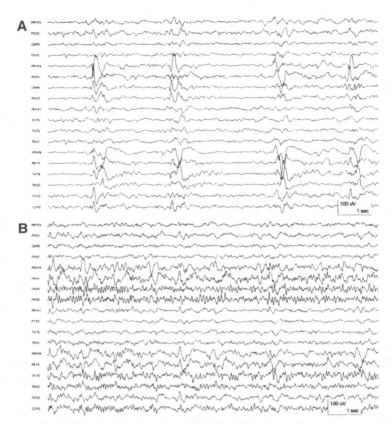

Fig. 3. Patient with nonconvulsive status epilepticus (NCSE). Reproduced from **Kaplan, PW.** 1999;16:341–352 with permission.

♦ First-line therapy for SE:
    – Overwhelming evidence exists in support of benzodiazepines (BDZ) being the rational first-line agent for the treatment of seizures that can be classified as SE
    – Although one well-conducted study supports the drug lorazepam as most efficacious, the three commonly used BDZs— (lorazepam, midazolam, and diazepam)—all are effective in appropriate doses (Table 6)
    – The advantage of Lorazepam is its long clinical duration of plasma concentration and action (1/2 15 h) secondary to its high water solubility, and slow elimination

Table 6
First-Line Therapy for SE

Benzodiazepine	Elimination time (t1/2 h)	Recommended dosage range
Lorazepam	15	0.05–0.1 mg/kg
Midazolam	2–4	0.05–0.2 mg/kg
Diazepam	20	0.1–0.4 mg/kg

Table 7
Second-Line Therpay for SE

2nd Line intravenous anticonvulsant	Dosage	Target serum level
Phenytoin (PHT)	15–20 mg/kg	15–20 mcg/mL
Fosphenytoin (fPHT)	15–20 mg/kg PE	15–20 mcg/mL
Valproate (VPA)	15–20 mg/kg	50–100 mcg/mL

– Diazepam is highly lipophilic, thus rapidly redistributing out of the plasma compartment. Thus its duration of action from a single bolus is quite brief (5–20 min)

– The elimination half-life (t1/2 20 h) of diazepam is the longest of the three, possibly contributing to prolonged sedation if large doses or infusions administered

– Midazolam is also lipophilic, very brief in action, yet rapidly metabolized yielding more consistent correlation between dosage and clearance

– Hence, if a continuous infusion of BDZs is desired, this latter drug offers the best pharmacokinetic profile

♦ Second-line therapy for SE:

– First-line BDZ treatment for SE is effective about 65% of the time in stopping SE

– For SE events that terminate using BDZ, the need for continued prophylaxis against seizures usually exists

– Intravenous agents are used for rapid effect and a fully awake patient is not required. BDZ are not appropriate agents for chronic use as single agents because of tachyphylaxis

– Phenytoin (PHT), fosphenytoin (fPHT), and sodium valproate (VPA) arecommon selections (Table 7)

– Although similar in parent compound, fPHT is a phosphate ester pro-drug of PHT

– fPHT is soluble in water and does not require an ethylene glycol vehicle as PHT. Consequently, it may be administered IV or IM. Since fPHT is metabolized to PHT in a few minutes, the drug is dosed as PHT equivalents (PE). FPHT can be administered 3 times faster than PHT (150 mg/min vs 50 mg/min). No hypotension from the ethylene glycol, but the required serum enzymatic conversion translates to similar kinetics of loading to target free serum PHT levels as the native compound

– When SE persists despite adequate trial of BDZ, the intravenous agents PHT/fPHT, and VPA are added to high-therapeutic target levels *Note: See* Table 8 for one commonly accepted algorithm

– As new anticonvulsants become available, their utility in treating refractory seizures and possibly SE has been evaluated, if only superficially

– Because of the lack of intravenous formulations, new drugs are assessed only as add-on agents

– There has been some success of these drugs (*see* Table 9) in the treatment of refractory seizures and may be used for SE in appropriate circumstances as patients are weaned from pharmacological EEG seizure suppression

– Because functional enteral absorption is required, deep pharmacologically-induced coma likely preclude such interventions

♦ Drug toxicity-induced SE: Need for nonconventional therapy:

– In certain circumstances of drug toxicity, specific therapies may be indicated. Most antibiotics that may cause seizures act via GABA antagonism

– Hence BDZ remain the first line therapy, and PHT and other agents may offer little added benefit

– In refractory cases or in other drug overdose states, hemodialysis is a viable therapeutic option

– Table 10 lists several more common drug offenders and potential treatment strategies

♦ Drug interactions:

Anticonvulsant drug interactions may complicate therapy for refractory SE where no single agent is able to control the seizures and poly-pharmacy is required

Table 8
Medical and Pharmacological Treatment for SE

Preserve airway and oxygenation by intubation. Order EEG to be available during therapy

Measure finger-stick blood glucose and administer iv glucose if less 40–60 mg/100 dL

Immediate benzodiazepines: IV lorazepam 5–10 mg, Diazepam 20–40 mg, or Midazolam 5–20 mg over 5 min

Phenytoin (PHT) loading dose 20 mg/kg at 50 mg/min or Fosphenytoin 20 mg/kg PE (PHT equivalents) at 150 mg/min. Goal serum level 15–20 mg/dL

Continuous EEG if available

If seizures continue phenytoin or fosphenytoin (additional 5–10 mg/kg or 5–10 mg/kg PE). Goal serum level 20–25 mg/dL

For refractory SE—Several options

Rapid pharmacological burst suppression/coma with hemodynamic support: Propofol 2 mg/kg and 150–200 mcg/kg/min infusion or thiopental 4 mg/kg and 0.3–0.4 mg/kg/min

Midazolam 0.2 mg/kg followed by 0.1–0.2 mg/kg/h may be used as alternative to propofol or thiopental

Valproate (VPA) 60–70 mg/kg may be tried

Pentobarbital 5–10 mg/kg followed by 1–10 mg/kg/h is common recipe for long term burst-suppression requirement

Weaning from EEG seizure suppression

Using continuous EEG, maintain in SE suppressed state (true burst-suppression may be, but not required) for 12–48 h before attempting to withdraw pharmacological coma

Ensure adequate anticonvulsant levels of selected agents for chronic seizure control. Aim for high- levels of fewest number of anticonvulsant agents. Most common: PHT and VPA

Wean infusion, follow EEG as background rhythm begins or increases. If break through seizures recur, re-bolus using 30–70% as necessary of original bolus amount required of infusion drug

Re-adjust anticonvulsant serum level or add additional agents before another wean attempt

Not uncommon for more than one adjustment to be made before successful wean

Adapted from **Varelas P and Mirski MA**, 2001.

225

Table 9
Indications for Newer Anticonvulsant Drugs As Adjunctive Therapy for Refractory Seizures

	Primary generalized	*Partial*
Lamotrigine	Yes	Yes
Gabapentin		Yes
Felbamate[a]	Yes	Yes
Topiramate		Yes
Tiagabine		Yes
Vigabatrin[b]	Yes	Yes

[a]Restricted use because of aplastic anemia
[b]Not available in the United States
Adapted from **Varelas P and Mirski MA.**, 2001.

Table 10
Therapies for Specific Drug-Induced SE

Drug precipitating SE	*Treatment options*
Antibiotics: Penicillins, B-Lactams, Fluoroquinolones	BDZ, Hemodialysis
Theophylline	Midazolam, Hemodialysis
Isoniazid	Intravenous Pyridoxine

Adapted from **Varelas P and Mirski MA.** , 2001.

– Usually this occurs when weaning from EEG suppressive therapy (e.g., barbiturates, propofol) is undertaken
– The desire is to wean with maximal serum level of a single selected anticonvulsant (i.e., PHT or VPA)
– Despite attaining high levels, break through seizures persist
– It is important to recognize that anticonvulsants may stimulate hepatic enzyme systems or alter serum protein binding, thereby disturbing the kinetics of other agents
– Table 11 describes the common know effects of anticonvulsants on each other
– Similarly, anticonvulsants may interact with common drugs used in the ICU setting where patients treated for SE are commonly managed
– Table 12 describes the alterations in efficacy of several commonly used medications

Table 11
Alteration in Drug-Plasma Levels With Combination Anticonvulsants

		Effect on plasma levels of primary agents				
Added Drug	*% bound*	*PHT*	*PB*	*CBZ*	*VPA*	*BDZ*
PHT	90		~	↓	↓	
PB	45	_, then ↓		~	↓	↓
CBZ	75	~		~	↓	↓	↓
VPA	90	↓ *	↑	~ or ↑ **		↑
BDZ		↓		~		~

Abbr: % bound, percentage serum protein bound; PHT, phenytoin; PB, phenobarbital; CBZ, carbamazepine; VPA, valproate; BDZ, benzodiazepines; ↓, decrease; ↑, increase; ~, variable; *, ↑ free DPH level; **, epoxide.
Adapted from **Varelas P and Mirski MA.**, 2001.

Table 12
Effects of Anticonvulsant Drugs on Commonly Used Medications

	Effect on plasma levels or clinical effectiveness of primary agents				
Added drug	*Warfarin*	*Theophylline*	*Steroids*	*Haloperidol*	*Lithium*
PHT	↓	↓	↓		
PB	↓	↓	↓	↓	
CBZ	↓	↓	↓	↓	↑

Abbr: PHT, phenytoin; P, Phenobarbital; CBZ, carbamazepine; ↓, decrease; ↓, increase
Adapted from **Varelas P and Mirski MA.**, 2001.

Key Points

♦ GCSE is rapidly assessed and treated to prevent further primary and secondary brain injury and systemic manifestations of muscle convulsive activity and risk of cardiopulmonary complications
♦ Intubation is suggested as nearly all AEDs have sedative effects compounding coma from SE
♦ Treatable causes of SE should be identified early
♦ An algorithm should be followed with sequential drug administration for persistent SE

♦ NCSE may not need as aggressive treatment as GCSE
♦ EEG is recommended to determine resolution of SE or presence of nonclinical SE

Suggested Reading

Bleck TP. Management approaches to prolonged status epilepticus. *Epilepsia* 1999;40(S1):S59-S63.

Brenner RP. Is it status? *Epilepsia* 2002;43(S3):S103–S113.

Coulter DA and DeLorenzo RJ. Basic mechanisms of status epilepticus. *Adv Neurol* 1999;79:725–733.

Kaplan PW. Assessing the outcomes in patients with nonconvulsive status epilepticus: nonconvulsive status epilepticus is undersiagnosed, potentially overtreated, and confounded by morbidity. *J Clin Neurophysiol* 1999;16:341–352.

Lowenstein DH. Status epilepticus: An overview of the clinical problem. *Epilepsia* 1999;40 (S1):S3–S8.

Niedermeyer E. Epileptic seizure disorders. In: *Electroencephalography: Basic Principles, Clinical Applications, and Related Fields.* (Niedermeyer E and Lopes da Silva F eds.), Baltimore: Williams and Wilkins; 1993:461–565.

Treiman DM, et. al. Acomparison of four treatments for generalized convulsive status epilepticus. *NEJM* 1998;339:792–798.

Wasterlain CG, Fujikawa DG, Penix L, and Sankar R. Pathophysiological mechanisms of brain damage from status epilepticus. *Epilepsia* 1993;34(S1):S37–S53.

Varelas P and Mirski MA. Seizures in the ICU. *J. Neurosurg. Anesthesiol.* 2001;13:163–175.

16 Blood Pressure Management

Michel T. Torbey

Concepts of Autoregulation and Cerebral Perfusion Pressure

♦ The central nervous system (CNS) is susceptible to extremes in blood pressure fluctuations. On one extreme, hypertension is associated with increased risk of bleeding and increased cerebral edema; on another extreme hypotension is associated with watershed infarcts or global cerebral ischemia

♦ Cerebral blood flow (CBF) is relatively constant over a wide range of systemic blood pressure (BP) or cerebral perfusion pressures (CPP) in healthy normal brain

♦ Continuous measurement of CBF is difficult. Thus CPP provides a bedside guide to assess the adequacy of cerebral perfusion

♦ Normal values for CPP are between 70 and 100 mmHg.

♦ Autoregulation is usually preserved in uncomplicated arterial hypertension. But the autoregulatory curve is shifted toward higher values of arterial pressure

♦ Clinical consequence of the upward shift is that, if BP in a hypertensive patient is reduced rapidly to low-normal values, symptoms and signs of cerebral ischemia may occur at arterial pressures that are well tolerated by normotensive patients

♦ Choice of anti-hypertensive agent is important because some agents, in addition to their antihypertensive effect, may affect or abolish CBF autoregulation, making the acute lowering of arterial pressure even more hazardous

From: *Current Clinical Neurology: Handbook of Neurocritical Care*
Edited by: A. Bhardwaj, M. A. Mirski, and J. A. Ulatowski © Humana Press Inc., Totowa, NJ

Antihypertensive Agents

♦ Several classes of pharmacological agents can be used in critically ill neurologic patients for the treatment of hypertension (*see* Table 1)

♦ An ideal agent in the ICU environment is easily titratable, given parenterally with minimal side effects, and has a short duration of action

♦ Other important therapeutic considerations include effects on cerebral autoregulation, regional CBF, and intracranial pressure (ICP)

Vasopressor agents

♦ Table 2 summarizes the most common agents that have minimal or no effect on cerebral vessels and hence are most frequently utilized for BP augmentation in critically ill neurologic patients (e.g., vasospasm following subarachnoid hemorrhage [SAH] and, more recently, ischemic stroke)

♦ Choice of a suitable pressor agent depends on its cardiac, systemic effect profile, and the patient's general medical condition. Phenylephrine or norepinephrine are used to augment BP in patients with preserved left-ventricular function, whereas patients with low-cardiac function may require inopressors like dopamine or epinephrine

Approach to Hypertension in Acute Neurological Disorders

♦ Subarachnoid hemorrhage (SAH):
  – Hypertension is often present immediately following aneurysmal rupture but may not require treatment in all patients
  – Current early treatment of SAH includes analgesia and sedation, anticonvulsant therapy (IV phenytoin) and central calcium channel antagonist (nimodipine) all of which can help lower BP
  – Hypertension in the setting of SAH may represent a "hyperadrenergic" state or a "Cushing's" reflex. Thus, it is important to recognize if BP elevation is associated with increased ICP
  – Maintenance of CPP > 70 mmHg is paramount to avoid exacerbation of cerebral ischemia in patients with intracranial hypertension
  – Figure 1 outlines the guidelines used for BP management in SAH

♦ Intracerebral hemorrhage:
  – BP management is of particular importance in hypertensive intracerebral hemorrhage (ICH)

Table 1
Common Antihypertensive Agents Used in Neurologically Ill Patients

Medication	Mechanism of action	Bolus dose	Infusion rate	Pros	Cons
Labetalol	$\alpha_1, \beta_1, \beta_2$ receptor antagonist	5–20 mg IV q 15 min for a total of 340 mg	0.5–2 mg/min	Rapid onset of action No effect on ICP	CHF Bronchospasm Bradycardia Hypoglycemia
Esmolol	β_1-selective	500 µg/kg over 1 min	50–200 µg/kg/min	Rapid onset of action No effect on ICP	Bradycardia CHF
Enalaprilat	ACE inhibitor	0.625–5 mg IV q6 h	No drip	No effect on ICP or CBF	Could cause abrupt decrease in BP Potential ↑ ICP in patients with poor compliance Renal dysfunction
Hydralazine	Vasodilator	2.5–10 mg IV Q20–30 min for a max of 40 mg	No drip	Good antihypertensive effect	Longer duration of action ↑CBF, ↑ ICP, reflex tachcardia Glomerulonephritis, Lupus like syndrome, hemolytic anemia (chronic use)
Nitroglycerin	Vasodilator	50 mcg IV	5–100 ug/kg/min	Short duration of action Rapid onset of action	↑ CBF, ↑ICP Methemoglobin production ↓CBF
Clonidine	α_2-agonist	0.1–0.2 mg PO	No drip	Might be helpful in alcohol withdrawal	Sedation Rebound hypertension Hypotension
Nicardipine	Ca^{++} channel antagonist	No bolus	5 mg/h, up to 15 mg/h increase by 1–2.5 mg/h Q15 min	Rapid onset of action Tritratable	Reflex tachycardia

Abbr: ACE, Angiotensin converting enzyme

Table 2
Common Vasopressor Agents Used in Neurologically Ill Patients

Medication	Mechanism of action	Infusion rate	Adverse Effects
Phenylephrine	α_1-receptor agonist	Initial 40 µg/min Max 200 µg/min	A-V shunting Tachyphylaxis
Norepinephrine	α- and β_1-receptor agonist ($\alpha > \beta$)	Initial 1 µg/min Max 40 µg/min	Visceral and extremities hypoperfusion
Epinephrine	α- and β-receptor agonist ($\beta > \alpha$)	Initial 2 µg/min Max 20 µg/min	Tachyarryrythmia
Dopamine	D1-receptor agonist (at lower doses) α_1- and β_1-receptor agonist (at higher doses)	Initial 1 µg/kg/min Initial 1 µg/kg/min Max 40 µg/kg/min	Coronary ischemia
Dobutamine	α- and β-receptor agonist ($\beta > \alpha$)	Initial 0.5 µg/kg/min Max 40 µg/Kg/min	Tachyarrhythmia

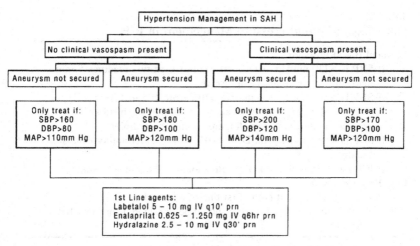

Fig. 1. Blood pressure management in SAH.

- Persistent bleeding is more likely to occur if the BP remains significantly elevated. Thus effective control of BP has potential benefits
- Optimal level of a patient's BP should be based on individual factors such as chronic hypertension, elevated ICP, age, presumed cause of ICH, and interval since onset
- Careful clinical neurological monitoring is still essential during the treatment of hypertension to ensure that this does not result in cerebral hypoperfusion and consequent secondary ischemic brain injury
- Table 3 provides recommendations and guidelines by the American Heart Association (AHA) for management of BP in patients with ICH
♦ Ischemic stroke:
- Most stroke patients are moderately to severely hypertensive at onset, probably as a result of compensatory central mechanism designed to maintain cerebral perfusion
- Optimal management of elevated BP is still a common clinical concern in acute stroke. Initial approach to BP management in stroke patients who are not candidates for thrombolytic therapy is to first observe patients for stress, control vomiting, and ensure that the bladder is emptied

Table 3
Guidelines to Blood Pressure Mangement in ICH

Elevated Blood Pressure
    –If SBP is >230 mmHg or DBP >140 mmHg on two readings 5 min
      apart, institute sodium nitroprusside
    –If SBP is from 180 to 230 mmHg, DBP from 105 to 140 mm Hg, or
      MAP ≥ 130 mmHg on two readings 20 min apart, institute
      intravenous labetalol, esmolol, enalaprilat, Nicardipine
    –If SBP is <180 mmHg and DBP <105 mmHg, defer antihypertensive
      therapy
    –If ICP monitoring is available, CPP should be kept at >70 mmHg
Low Blood Pressure
    –Volume replenishment is the first line of approach
    –If hypotension persists, pressors should be considered for low SBP
      < 90 mmHg

Adapted from **Broderick et al.**, 1999.

    – Based on the AHA recommendations, treatment with anti-
hypertensive agents should be avoided unless BP is profoundly
elevated (systolic blood pressure [SBP] > 220 mmHg, mean arterial pressure [MAP] < 130 mmHg)
    – If the patient has other medical conditions such as acute
myocardial ischemia or evidence of hemorrhagic transformation
of the cerebral infarct, the recommendation is modified to maintain SBP <170 mm Hg
    – Use of sublingual nifedipine is strongly discouraged because
of potential excessive and precipitous lowering of BP. In patients
who are candidates for rtPA, recommendations of the NINDS
rt-PA study group should be followed (*see* Table 4)
♦ Other neurological disorders:
    – Patients following carotid endarterectomy should be treated
aggressively to lower their MAP to 80–100 mmHg. Our experience indicates that these patients have an exaggerated bradycardic
response with β-blockers and hence hydralazine or enalaprilat is a
better choice agent. Occasionally nitrates (IV) are needed
    – Spinal cord injury: MAP should be maintained 80–100 mmHg
to prevent hypoperfusion of the spinal cord. Calcium channel
antagonists are first choice agents. α-receptor blockers are the
second choice of agents

Table 4
NINDS rt-PA Study Group Guidelines to Blood Pressure Management in Ischemic Stroke

Pretreatment
  –Monitor BP every 15 min and observe for BP >184/110 mm Hg
  –If BP is >185/110 mmHg, institute Nitroglycerine paste or labetalol,
    Nicardipine
  –If BP persists >185/110 mmHg, do not treat with rt-PA
Intratreatment and Posttreatment
  –Monitor BP every 15 min for 2 h, every 30 min for 6 h, every 60 min
    for 16 h
  –If DBP >140 mm Hg, institute iv nitroprusside
  –If SBP >230 mmHg and/or DBP 121–140 mmHg, institute labetalol,
    Nicardipine
  –If SBP 180–230 Hg and/or DBP 105–120 mmHg on two readings
    5–10 min apart, institute labetalol, Nicardipine
  –Monitor BP every 15 min during antihypertensive therapy and observe
    for hypotension

Adapted from **Adams et al.**, 1996.

– Hypertensive encephalopathy (HE): goal is to gradually decrease the MAP by approx 25% or to reduce the diastolic blood pressure (DBP) to approx 100 mmHg over a period of several minutes to hours. Precipitous reduction in BP to normotensive or hypotensive level should be avoided, as it may provoke cerebral hypoperfusion. Sodium nitroprusside is the drug of choice for the initial treatment of HE. Other agents such as β-blockers or ACE-inhibitors should be used after initial control of BP. Hydralazine appears to be less effective in treating HE. Bed rest, sedation and analgesia may further help BP control

– Traumatic brain injury (TBI): cardiovascular abnormalities such as elevated BP, cardiac output, and tachycardia are frequently encountered. These findings are typical of a hyperadrenergic state, and should not be confused with Cushing's triad of bradycardia, bradypnea, and hypertension. β-adrenergic blocking agents are recommended for treatment of hypertension after head injury, especially in patients with hyperadrenergic condition

– Guillain-Barre syndrome (GBS): hypertension and tachycardia are best left untreated because they are only transient, and β-blockade and antihypertensive treatment may aggravate incipient bradycardia or hypotension. However, older patients with coronary heart disease must be treated. Use of vasoactive medications should be done with caution, and preferably medications with a short half-life in the ICU setting. If there is evidence of cardiac decompensation, or other end-organ injury or MAP exceeds 120 mmHg, then sodium nitroprusside should be administered cautiously

Therapeutic Hypertension

♦ Although hypertension may exacerbate brain injury in patients with ICH or stroke, in certain clinical situations it may have some therapeutic role

♦ Patients with ischemic stroke secondary to large vessel occlusive disease with poor collaterals and who are not candidates for rtPA may benefit from BP augmentation

♦ In SAH, hypervolemic, hypertensive therapy is the cornerstone of medical management in patients with symptomatic vasospasm following aneurysmal SAH. Although this therapeutic strategy has never been validated in a large randomized controlled trial, several uncontrolled series have reported the beneficial effects of BP augmentation in this subset of patients

♦ Figure 2 describes the algorithm used in patients with SAH or stroke

Key Points

♦ Basic principles of BP management in critically ill neurologic patients include:
- To ameliorate systemic hypertension
- To avoid systemic hypotension
- Maintain adequate BP and CPP, thereby avoiding secondary brain and spinal cord injury
- Utilizing agents that have minimal effects on ICP and CBF autoregulation
- CPP should be maintained >70 mmHg
- Reduction of CPP below 70 mmHg can trigger reflex vasodilatation and ICP elevation
- If CPP is <70 mmHg and ICP is >20 mmHg, elevation of MAP (and thus CPP) with a vasopressor may lead to a reflex reduction of ICP by reducing cerebral vasodilatation (and thus cerebral blood volume) that occurs in response to inadequate perfusion

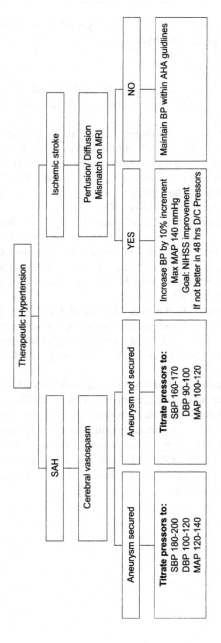

Fig. 2. Hypertensive therapy in SAH and stroke patients.

- Favorable agents for treatment of hypertension include labetalol, enalaprilat, and hydralazine

Suggested Reading

Paulson OB, Waldemar G, Schmidt JF, and Strandgaard S. Cerebral circulation under normal and pathologic conditions. *Am J Cardiol* 1989;63(6):2C–5C.

Kassell NF, Peerless SJ, Durward QJ et al. Treatment of ischemic deficits from vasospasm with intravascular volume expansion and induced arterial hypertension. *Neurosurgery* 1982;11(3):337–343.

Kassell NF, Torner JC, Haley EC, Jr., et al. The International Cooperative Study on the Timing of Aneurysm Surgery. Part 1: overall management results. *J Neurosurg* 1990;73(1):18–36.

Broderick JP, Adams HP, Jr., Barsan W, et al. Guidelines for the management of spontaneous intracerebral hemorrhage: a statement for healthcare professionals from a special writing group of the Stroke Council, American Heart Association. *Stroke* 1999;30(4):905–915.

Britton M and Carlsson A. Very high blood pressure in acute stroke. *J Intern Med* 1990;228(6):611–615.

Adams HP, Jr., Brott TG, Crowell RM, et al. Guidelines for the management of patients with acute ischemic stroke. A statement for healthcare professionals from a special writing group of the Stroke Council, American Heart Association [see comments]. *Stroke* 1994;25(9): 1901–1914.

Adams HP, Jr., Brott TG, Furlan AJ, et al. Guidelines for thrombolytic therapy for acute stroke: a supplement to the guidelines for the management of patients with acute ischemic stroke. A statement for healthcare professionals from a Special Writing Group of the Stroke Council, American Heart Association. *Circulation* 1996;94(5):1167–1174.

Rordorf G, Cramer SC, Efird JT, et al. Pharmacological elevation of blood pressure in acute stroke. Clinical effects and safety. *Stroke* 1997;28(11):2133–2138.

17 Airway Management

Lauren Berkow

Patients Potentially Requiring Airway Management

♦ Patients with low Glasgow Coma Score (GCS) < 8–9
♦ Closed head injury
♦ Spinal cord injury
♦ Subarachnoid or intracranial hemorrhage (SAH or ICH)
♦ Myasthenia Gravis (MG) crisis
♦ Guillain–Barré syndrome
♦ Acute stroke (large hemispheric, basilar artery thrombosis)
♦ Combative patients requiring a procedure (computerized tomography [CT], magnetic resonance imaging [MRI], angiography)
♦ Patients at high-risk for aspiration
♦ Patients with low GCS
♦ Meets intubation criteria

Basic Intubation Criteria

♦ Respiratory rate greater than 30 breaths per minute
♦ Tidal volume less than 10 cc per kilogram
♦ Significant desaturations by pulse oximetry on maximum supplemental oxygen
♦ P_aCO_2 greater than 60 mmHg on arterial blood gas (ABG) (unless patient with compensated chronic obstructive pulmonary disease [COPD])
♦ P_aO_2 <70 mmHg on 40% oxygen
♦ Inability to protect airway (i.e., aspiration, obtundation, trauma, obstruction)
♦ Significant muscle weakness affecting respiratory muscles (Negative Inspiratory Force (NIF) < –25 cm H_2O. Vital capacity (VC) < 15 mL/kg)

From: *Current Clinical Neurology: Handbook of Neurocritical Care*
Edited by: A. Bhardwaj, M. A. Mirski, and J. A. Ulatowski © Humana Press Inc., Totowa, NJ

Medications Used for Intubation
(at discretion of intubating personnel,
none or some from each group may be chosen)

♦ Sedating agents (lower doses usually required in patients with severe brain injury):
- Benzodiazepines: Midazolam, 0.01–0.10 mg/kg
- Narcotics: Fentanyl, 1–3 µg/kg
- Thiopental: 2–4 mg/kg , usually administered by anesthesia personnel
- Propofol: 1–2 mg/kg,usually administered by anesthesia personnel
- Etomidate: 0.2 mg/kg, usually administered by anesthesia personnel
♦ Paralytic agents:
- Succinylcholine :
  • Short acting, effective within 30 s, does not require reversal of paralysis with additional medication, lasts 3–5 min, dose 1–1.5 mg/kg
  • Use only if emergent. Risk of hyperkalemia
- Longer acting muscle relaxants (i.e., Vecuronium, Rocuronium, Pancuronium):
  • These have longer delay to onset of paralysis, require reversal of paralysis with additional medications, average duration 30–90 min

Tools Required for Intubation

♦ Personnel skilled in endotracheal intubation (i.e., anesthesiologist, intensivist, emergency room physician)
♦ Mechanical ventilator, respiratory therapy present or en route
♦ Intravenous access to administer medications
♦ Continuous monitoring of vital signs, including pulse oximetry
♦ End-tidal carbon dioxide monitoring if available to confirm intubation
♦ 100% Oxygen by mask
♦ Suction
♦ Medications for intubation and resuscitation
♦ Endotracheal tubes (ETT) of various sizes and stylette (most common 7.0 ETT in females and 8.0 ETT in males)

♦ Laryngoscopy blades of various sizes. Most common are Macintosh 3 and 4, Miller 2 and 3
♦ Tape to secure endotracheal tube. Avoid circumferential taping that may occlude jugular blood flow raising intracranial pressure (ICP).
♦ 10-cc syringe to inflate cuff of tube
♦ Access to head of bed and patient. Often difficult in intensive care setting
♦ Post-intubation confimatory chest radiograph

Conditions Often Associated With Difficult Intubation (Fig. 1)

♦ Previous history of difficult intubation
♦ Achondroplasia
♦ Unstable cervical spine, especially C1–C3
♦ Morbid obesity
♦ Rheumatoid arthritis, especially if chin-on-chest deformity present
♦ Ankylosing spondylitis
♦ Significantly decreased neck range of motion
♦ Obstructive sleep apnea, especially if continuous positive airway pressure (CPAP) required
♦ Significant micrognathia
♦ Facial trauma
♦ Acromegaly

Basic Extubation Criteria

♦ Respiratory rate less than 30 breaths per minute
♦ Tidal volume 10 cc per kilogram or greater
♦ ABG parameters within normal limits, specifically lack of hypercarbia or hypoxemia
♦ Minimal supplemental oxygen requirements (40% O_2 or less)
♦ Good muscle strength, able to follow commands, lift head for five seconds
♦ Able to protect airway, bulbar muscles, gag reflex intact
♦ GCS ≥ 8. Cognitive airway protection
♦ Stable hemodynamics, no inotropic support
♦ Reversal of muscle blocking drugs if needed
♦ All sedatives and narcotics should be held for 2 h prior to extubation

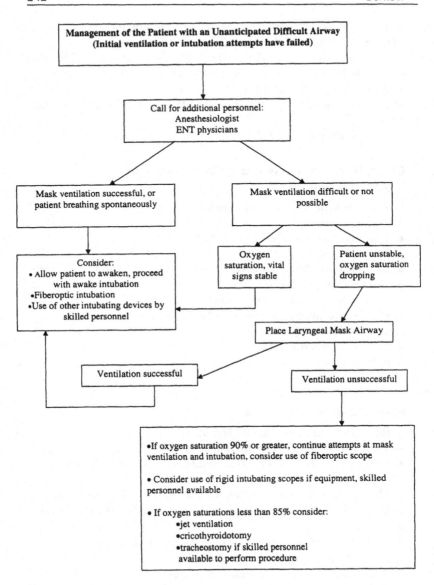

Fig. 1.

Airway Management of the Patient With a Full Stomach or Risk of Aspiration

♦ Decompress stomach if possible prior to intubation. If not possible, decompress stomach immediately after intubation

♦ If no contra-indications, administer Ranitidine (50 mg) and Metoclopramide (10 mg) IV (must be given 10–30 min in advance)

♦ Avoid medications that increase secretions, such as ketamine

♦ Administer cricoid pressure (pressure over the trachea in the neck that compresses the esophagus) to lessen aspiration of stomach contents during intubation

♦ Avoid mask ventilation prior to intubation ("rapid sequence" intubation) unless absolutely necessary

♦ Use short-acting, quick-onset medications, if any, to provide rapid intubating conditions. Most common: succinylcholine 1.0–1.5 mg/kg, etomidate, propofol or thiopental

♦ Maintain cricoid pressure during any mask ventilation and until *after* tube placement is *confirmed* by bilateral breath sounds on auscultation and end-tidal CO_2

♦ Consider awake intubation to avoid need for sedation or mask ventilation, allow for maintenance of airway reflexes. May require elective fiberoptic assistance

Management of the Patient With a Known or Suspected Difficult Airway

♦ Consider early airway intervention if progression of symptoms suspected to avoid need for emergent intubation

♦ Have physician(s) skilled in difficult airway management available, consider arranging for ENT physician back-up

♦ Consider awake intubation techniques to avoid need for sedation and mask ventilation

♦ Consider use of special airway equipment:
  – Fiberoptic scope for nasal or oral intubation
  – Light wand stylette: blind technique, light used to guide tube into trachea
  – Eschmann Stylette: helpful when cords anterior or not visualized
  – Laryngeal mask airway (LMA): helpful when mask ventilation difficult or not possible

♦ Have medications available to topicalize airway, consider IV glycopyrrolate to decrease airway secretions

♦ If general anesthetic given, confirm mask ventilation *prior* to administration of neuromuscular blocking drugs

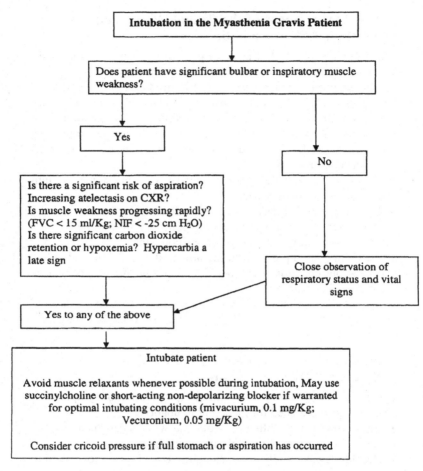

Fig. 2.

Myasthenia Gravis (*see* Fig. 2)

♦ Bulbar muscle weakness may lead to respiratory distress, aspiration
♦ Weakness of respiratory muscles may also lead to respiratory insufficiency
♦ Very sensitive to narcotics. May lead to hypoventilation and need for airway management
♦ Often require mechanical ventilation postoperatively or during acute crisis
♦ Intubation should be considered early if weakness progressing

Extubation of the Myasthenia Gravis Patient

♦ Muscle weakness improved, patient stable
♦ Adequate vital signs (NIF, FVC, RR), no hypercarbia or hypoxemia present on minimal oxygen supplementation (≤40%)
♦ If muscle relaxants used during mechanical ventilation, confirm full reversal (twitch monitor, five second head lift, minimal ventilator settings)
♦ Hold all sedatives, especially narcotics
♦ Confirm presence of strong cough and gag reflex, minimal secretions
♦ Anticipate possible need for re-intubation, ensure all necessary personnel and equipment readily available

Guillain–Barré Syndrome

♦ May require ventilation if respiratory muscles involved
♦ Sudden respiratory insufficiency may occur if paralysis rapidly progressive
♦ Succinylcholine should be avoided if muscle paralysis required because of risk of hyperkalemia
♦ Sensitivity to other muscle relaxants varies widely from hypersensitivity to resistance
♦ Hemodynamic changes may be significant during intubation because of autonomic nervous system dysfunction:
   – Hypotension after sedation or intubation
   – Hypertension and tachycardia during intubation because of noxious stimulation
♦ Vital signs should be closely monitored and treated aggressively during and after intubation
♦ Consider extubation after extubation criteria are met and respiratory and muscle strength is returning

Airway Management Issues in Rheumatoid Arthritis

♦ Unstable cervical spine may be present:
   – Atlanto-occipital instability
   – Significant cervical myelopathy
   – Significant spinal cord compression
♦ Muscle weakness may lead to chin-on-chest deformity or inability to straighten or move neck. May result in difficult ventilation and intubation
♦ Chronic steroid use may cause skin and mucosal fragility, leading to increased risk of bleeding or bruising during intubation

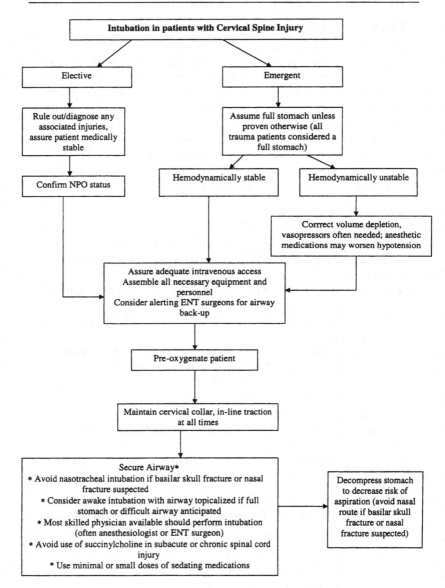

Fig. 3.

♦ Felty's syndrome (low platelet count) may also cause increased risk of bleeding

♦ HALO placement may be required for spine stability, thus limiting access to airway as well as restricting neck mobility

♦ Laryngeal, arytenoid cartilage arthritis may necessitate use of smaller endotracheal tube

♦ Temporomandubular joint dysfunction (TMJ) disease may limit mouth opening, making intubation difficult

Cerebrovascular Accident (CVA)

♦ May require intubation if:
  − Risk of aspiration –Low GCS score (≤8 common threshold for loss of airway protection)
  − Combative because of altered mental status; requires deep sedation for bedside care
  − Requires sedation or airway protection for procedure (CT, MRI, angiography)

♦ Consider hyperventilation if increased intracranial pressure present

♦ May be anticoagulated, increasing the risk of bleeding during intubation

♦ If CVA severe, may require prolonged intubation and tracheostomy

♦ Cranial nerve paresis may lead to laryngospasm (CN X) or aspiration (CN IX)

Airway Management for Patients With Intracerebral Aneursysms

♦ Hunt–Hess grade 3 or higher may need intubation for airway protection

♦ Aneursyms of any grade will need intubation for clipping or coiling

♦ May require short-term hyperventilation if increased intracranial pressure present

♦ Intubation should proceed after adequate sedation or general anesthesia to avoid rupture of aneursym

♦ Blood pressure should be adequately controlled during and after intubation

♦ Airway manipulation should be avoided in unruptured or low-grade ruptured aneurysms unless absolutely necessary

♦ If hypothermia or burst suppression used intra-operatively, may require post-operative mechanical ventilation

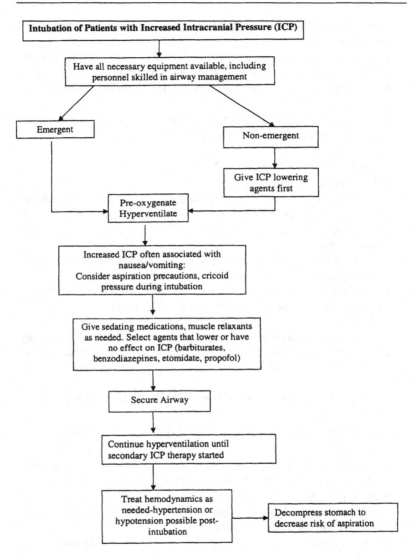

Fig. 4.

♦ If increased intracranial pressure (ICP) present, follow the intubation algorithm for increased ICP (Fig. 4)

Pituitary Tumors

♦ Patients with acromegaly often present with a difficult airway:
- Large tongue and jaw lead to difficulty in ventilation
- Patients may develop sleep apnea because of enlargement of airway tissue
- Vocal cords may be difficult to visualize because of soft tissue edema

♦ Chronic steroid use may lead to Cushingoid appearance, airway edema

♦ Electrolyte abnormalities may lead to hemodynamic arrhythmias during intubation

♦ Transsphenoidal surgery requires entry through the cribiform plate to the pituitary gland:
- Avoid nasotracheal intubation after surgery
- Avoid use of continuous positive airway pressure (CPAP) after surgery
- Patients with sleep apnea may require post-operative intubation until CPAP can be resumed
- Airway edema may develop intra-operatively as a result of head-down position during surgery

Key Points

♦ Airway management may be necessary to protect the lungs because of reflexes in coma or brainstem injury or to protect an agitated brain-injured patient and bedside personnel

♦ Special intubation caution is needed in patients with elevated ICP and neuromuscular disorders

♦ Intubation and extubation criteria depend on mental status examination and status of neuromuscular strength

♦ Certain neurologic conditions present specific needs in airway management (i.e., ICP, neck instability, untreated aneurysm)

♦ Neurologic conditions may be associated with head and neck fractures

♦ Always have adequate personnel and equipment for difficult airway management

Suggested Reading

Practice Guidelines for management of the difficult airway: an updated report by the ASA Task Force on management of the difficult airway. *Anesthesiology* 2003;98:1269–1277.

Schmitt H, Buchfelder M, Radespiel-Trager M, Fahlbusch R. Difficult intubation in acromegalic patients. *Anesthesiology* 2000;93(1): 110–114.

18 Analgesia, Sedation, and Paralysis in the Neuro-Intensive Care Unit

Mitzi K. Hemstreet

Analgesia in the Neuro-Intensive Care Unit (ICU)

- ◆ Indications:
  - – Postoperative pain
  - – Traumatic injury
  - – Subacute or chronic pain
- ◆ General precautions:
  - – Equipment and personnel to intubate and mechanically ventilate must be readily available with use of narcotic agonists
  - – Decreased level-of-consciousness or obtundation
  - – Poor airway protection
  - – Respiratory depression, hypercarbia, and increased intracranial pressure
  - – Impairment of neurological exam
  - – Hemodynamic instability
  - – Risk of bleeding dyscrasias with anti-platelet agents or nonsteroidal anti-inflammatory drugs (NSAIDs)
- ◆ Selected agents (many alternatives available):
  - – Narcotics:
    - • Fentanyl: Sublimaze
    - • Remifentanil: Ultiva
    - • Morphine
  - – NSAID:
    - • Ketorolac: Toradol
    - • Ibuprofen: Motrin

From: *Current Clinical Neurology: Handbook of Neurocritical Care*
Edited by: A. Bhardwaj, M. A. Mirski, and J. A. Ulatowski © Humana Press Inc., Totowa, NJ

Table 1
Properties of Selected Analgesics in the Neuro-ICU

Drug	Mechanism of action	Advantages	Disadvantages	Metabolism
Fentanyl (Sublimaze)	Narcotic agonist	Easily titrated, reversible with naloxone (Narcan)	Respiratory suppression, chest wall rigidity	Hepatic
Remifentanil (Ultiva)	Narcotic agonist	Easily titrated, reversible with naloxone (Narcan)	Respiratory suppression, chest wall rigidity	Plasma esterases
Morphine	Narcotic agonist	Reversible with naloxone (Narcan)	Respiratory suppression, longer duration of action	Hepatic (renal clearance of active metabolites)
Ketorolac (Toradol)	NSAID (nonspecific)	No respiratory suppression, intravenous	Risk of bleeding dyscrasias (1° GI, intracranial)	Hepatic (with renal clearance)
Ibuprofen (Motrin)	NSAID (nonspecific)	No respiratory suppression	Risk of bleeding dyscrasias (1° GI, intracranial)	Renal
Rofecoxib (Vioxx)	NSAID (selective COX-2 inhibitor)	No respiratory suppression, reduced risk of bleeding	Some risk of bleeding dyscrasias, only available in enteral form	Hepatic
Celecoxib (Celebrex)	NSAID (selective COX-2 inhibitor)	No respiratory suppression, reduced risk of bleeding	Some risk of bleeding dyscrasias, only available in enteral form	Hepatic

- Selective cyclo-oxygenase (COX-2) inhibitors:
  - Rofecoxib: Vioxx
  - Celecoxib: Celebrex

See Tables 1 and 2, and Fig. 1

Sedation in the Neuro-ICU

♦ Indications:
  - Agitation
  - Risk of self-injury or injury of others
  - Withdrawal from alcohol or drugs
  - Risk of self-extubation or removal of invasive monitors

Table 2
Administration of Selected Analgesics in the Neuro-ICU

Drug	Starting dose	Increase by	Maximum dose	Duration of action
Fentanyl (Sublimaze)	12.5–50 mcg IV every 20–30 min	12.5–50 mcg/ dose as needed	2–20 mcg/kg in 24 h (tolerance develops rapidly)	30–60 min after a single IV dose (longer for higher cumulative doses).
Remifentanil (Ultiva)	0.5–1.0 mcg/kg IV bolus	Infusion 0.025– 0.2 mcg/kg/min	0.2 mcg/kg/min	5–10 min after discontinuation of infusion.
Morphine	5–20 mg IM or 2–10 mg IV every 4 h	As needed for effect	Highly variable, tolerance develops within d	4–12 h (shortened by tolerance).
Ketorolac (Toradol)	15–60 mg IV or im every 6 h (decrease by ½ in those >65 yr old)	N/A	120 mg/d (60 mg/d for >65 yr old), Maximum duration of use is 5 d	4–12 h (increased in elderly and renal impairment).
Ibuprofen (Motrin)	400–800 mg PO every 6–8 h	N/A, single doses >400 mg not shown to have greater efficacy	1200–3200 mg in 24 h (higher dosages have increased risk of bleeding)	6–8 h
Rofecoxib (Vioxx)	12.5–25 mg PO every 24 h	As needed	50 mg in 24 h (max 5 d at this dose)	24–51 h
Celecoxib (Celebrex)	100–200 mg po every 12–24 h	As needed	400 mg in 24 h	12–33 h

- – Intracranial hypertension
- – Refractory systemic hypertension or sympathetic hyperactivity
- – Recurrent seizures or status epilepticus
- ♦ General precautions:
  - – Equipment and personnel to intubate and mechanically ventilate must be readily available
  - – Decreased level-of-consciousness or obtundation
  - – Poor airway protection

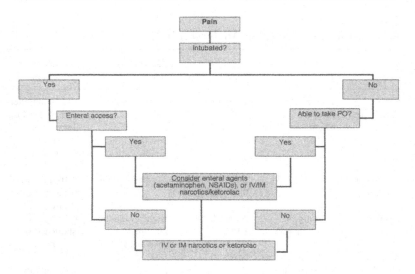

Fig. 1. Flow chart for pain management in the Neuro-ICU.

- Respiratory depression, hypercarbia, and increased intracranial pressure (ICP)
- Impairment of neurological exam
- Hemodynamic instability
♦ Selected agents (many alternatives available):
  - Narcotics:
    • Fentanyl
    • Remifentanil
    • Morphine
  - Benzodiazepines:
    • Lorazepam
    • Midazolam
    • Diazepam
  - Antihistamines:
    • Diphenhydramine
    • Hydroxyzin
  - Neuroleptics:
    • Haloperidol
    • Droperidol

– α-2 agonists:
- Clonidine
- Dexmedetomidine
– Propofol
– Barbiturates:
- Phenobarbital
- Pentobarbital
- Thiopental

See Tables 3 and 4, and Fig. 2

Paralysis in the Neuro-ICU

♦ Indications:
  – Facilitation of intubation
  – Brief bedside surgical procedures
  – Severe refractory intracranial hypertension
  – Severe pulmonary disease with inability to mechanically ventilate
♦ General Precautions:
  – Patient *must* be intubated with capacity to mechanically ventilate
  – Transient increase in ICP with depolarizing blockade (succinylcholine)
  – Unexpected prolongation of neuromuscular blockade (e.g., enzyme deficiencies, hepatic or renal dysfunction)
  – Complete loss of neurological examination
♦ Selected agents (many alternatives available):
  – Depolarizing neuromuscular blockade (e.g., succinylcholine)
  – Nondepolarizing neuromuscular blockers:
    - Pancuronium: Pavulon
    - Vecuronium: Norcuron
    - Rocuronium: Zemuron
  – Reversal of nondepolarizing neuromuscular blockers:
    - At least one twitch must be present by "train of four" monitoring before reversal is attempted
    - Neostigmine (acetylcholinesterase antagonist): 0.05–0.07 mg/kg IV, maximum 7 mg
    - Must be given with glycopyrrolate (to prevent excessive vagal tone): 0.01–0.014 mg/kg IV (give before neostigmine)

See Tables 5 and 6, and Fig. 3

Table 3
Properties of Selected Sedatives in the Neuro-ICU

Drug	Mechanism of action	Advantages	Disadvantages	Metabolism
Fentanyl (Sublimaze)	Narcotic agonist	Easily titrated, reversible with naloxone (Narcan)	Respiratory suppression, chest wall rigidity	Hepatic
Remifentanil (Ultiva)	Narcotic agonist	Easily titrated, reversible with naloxone (Narcan)	Respiratory suppression, chest wall rigidity	Plasma esterases
Morphine	Narcotic agonist	Reversible with naloxone (Narcan)	Respiratory suppression, longer duration of action	Hepatic (renal clearance of active metabolites)
Lorazepam (Ativan)	Benzodiazepine (intermediate)	Raises seizure threshold, reversible with flumazenil (Mazicon)	Respiratory depression, confusion	Hepatic
Midazolam (Versed)	Benzodiazepine (short-acting)	Easily-titrated, raises seizure threshold, reversible with flumazenil (Mazicon)	Respiratory depression, confusion	Hepatic
Diazepam (Valium)	Benzodiazepine (intermediate)	Raises seizure threshold, reversible with flumazenil (Mazicon)	Respiratory depression, confusion	Hepatic
Diphenhydramine (Benadryl)	Antihistamine/ Anticholinergic	No respiratory depression	Confusion, urinary retention (if patient's bladder not catheterized)	Hepatic
Hydroxyzine (Vistaril)	Antihistamine/ Anticholinergic	No respiratory depression	Confusion, somnolence	Hepatic
Haloperidol (Haldol)	Neuroleptic (dopamine antagonist)	No respiratory depression	May lower seizure threshold, movement disorders	Hepatic
Droperidol (Inapsine)	Neuroleptic (dopamine antagonist)	No respiratory depression	May lower seizure threshold, prolongs QT interval	Hepatic

(continued)

Table 3 *(continued)*

Drug	Mechanism of action	Advantages	Disadvantages	Metabolism
Clonidine (Catapres)	α-2 agonist	Reduces catecholamine hyperactivity in drug withdrawal and traumatic brain injury	Bradycardia, withdrawal hypertension	Hepatic and renal
Dexmedetomidine (Precedex)	α-2 agonist	Easily titrated, short duration, no respiratory depression	Bradycardia and either hypo- or hypertension (bolus dosing), limited to 24 h duration	Hepatic
Propofol (Diprivan)	Unknown (possible γ-aminobutyric acid [GABA] agonist)	Easily-titrated, lowers ICP	Respiratory suppression, hemodynamic instability, metabolic acidosis with prolonged use	Hepatic and extrahepatic
Phenobarbital (Luminal)	Barbiturate (enhances GABA activity)	Raises seizure threshold, lowers ICP	Respiratory suppression, hemodynamic instability	Hepatic
Pentobarbital (Nembutal)	Barbiturate (enhances GABA activity)	Raises seizure threshold, lowers ICP	Respiratory suppression, hemodynamic instability	Hepatic
Thiopental (Pentothal)	Barbiturate (enhances GABA activity)	Raises seizure threshold, lowers ICP	Respiratory suppression, hemodynamic instability	Hepatic

Table 4
Administration of Selected Sedatives in the Neuro-ICU

Drug	Starting dose	Increase by	Maximum dose	Duration of action
Fentanyl (Sublimaze)	Infusion 0.01–0.03 mcg/ kg/min (25–50 mcg/h, with or without bolus)	5–25 mcg/h every 15–30 min, up to 50– 200 mcg/h	Variable; above 200–300 mcg/h not recommended	30 min to h (increases with higher cumulative dose)
Remifentanil (Ultiva)	0.5–1.0 mcg/kg IV bolus	Infusion 0.025– 0.2 mcg/kg/min	0.2 mcg/kg/min	5–10 min after discontinuation of infusion
Morphine	2–10 mg IV every 4 h	As needed for effect	Highly variable; continuous infusion not recommended	4–12 h (shortened by tolerance).
Lorazepam (Ativan)	0.25–0.5 mg IV q 1–2 h	As needed for effect	4 mg in 8 h (higher for intubated patients)	6–8 h
Midazolam (Versed)	0.01–0.05 mg/kg (0.5–1 mg) IV every 5–30 min	Infusion 0.02– 0.1 mg/kg/h	Variable, but generally 0.1 mg/kg/h	2–6 h
Diazepam (Valium)	2–10 mg IV every 1–4 hrs	As needed for effect	30 mg in 24 h; active metabolites may accumulate	2–24 h (caused by redistribution from brain), but elimination takes days
Diphenhydramine (Benadryl)	25–50 mg IV every 6–8 h	As needed, up to 100 mg/dose	400 mg in 24 h	6–24 h
Hydroxyzine (Vistaril)	25–100 mg im every 4–6 h	As needed for effect	Variable, but generally <400 mg in 24 h	4–24 h
Haloperidol (Haldol)	0.5–5.0 mg IV im, or PO every 1 to 24 h	As needed for effect	Variable, but generally <20 mg in 24 h	4–24 h (after desirable effect is achieved)
Droperidol (Inapsine)	0.625 –2.5 mg IV every 4–24 h	Maximum additional doses of 1.25 mg	Variable, but generally <5 mg in 24 h	2–12 h
Clonidine (Catapres)	0.1 mg po every 8–24 h	Increase 0.1 mg/d every 1–2 d	0.6 mg/d	12–48 h (markedly prolonged in renal impairment)

(continued)

Table 4 *(continued)*

Drug	Starting dose	Increase by	Maximum dose	Duration of action
Dexmedetomidine (Precedex)	0.2–0.7 mcg/kg/h	0.1 mcg/kg/h every 5–10 min	0.7 mcg/kg/h for 24 h	2–6 h
Propofol (Diprivan)	25–50 mcg/kg/min	5–25 mcg/kg/min every 5–10 min	300 mcg/kg/min	15–30 min (increased to h with prolonged infusion)
Phenobarbital (Luminal)	1–3 mg/kg IV or IM (sedation); 15–20 mg/kg IV load (status epilepticus)	Titration based on plasma levels; 30–200 mg/d divided every 8–24 h	Up to 200 mg in 24 h (after loading dose)	10–24 h (although elimination may take up to 120 h)
Pentobarbital (Nembutal)	3–30 mg/kg IV (loading for refractory intracranial HTN or status epilepticus)	Infusion 1–2 mg/kg/h, titrate to plasma levels and burst-suppression by electroencephalo-cardiogram (EEG)	Highly variable, but generally <2400 mg in 24 h after loading dose	Highly variable; 3–4 h, although elimination may take 50–150 h after steady state
Thiopental (Pentothal)	1–5 mg/kg IV (intubation or acute Tx of seizures or elevated ICP)	Repeat as necessary; continuous infusion rate highly variable	Highly variable, based on hemodynamic tolerance and desired effects	Min (caused by redistribution from brain); elimination takes 8–24 h, and duration is prolonged with repeated dosing

Key Points

♦ Preservation of the neurologic exam is paramount when considering choice of analgesics, sedatives, and paralytics. As such, shorter acting and reversible agents are preferable

♦ Neuro-ICU patients often have poor airway protection due to underlying neurologic pathology (even when awake and alert)

♦ Patients with pre-existent neurologic impairment are more sensitive to the sedative effects of multiple medications, and may take a prolonged time to awaken from sedation or general anesthesia

♦ Patients with traumatic brain injury may show sympathetic hyperactivity that requires treatment with multiple agents

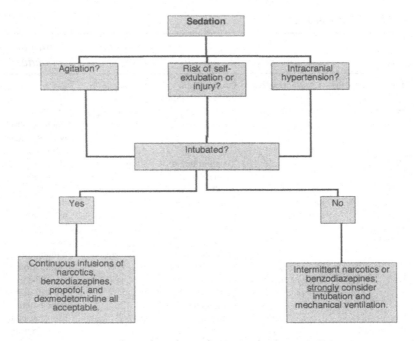

Fig. 2. Flow chart for sedation in the Neuro-ICU.

♦ Patients undergoing drug and alcohol withdrawal may also show sympathetic hyperactivity. However, an acute change in mental status (including agitation) may be caused by worsening intracranial pathology, which must be ruled out

♦ The cause of any acute change in mental status must be investigated for new intracranial pathology, metabolic or toxic disarray, infection, or adverse reaction to medications before being treated symptomatically

♦ Any medication that impairs respiratory drive may lead to hypercarbia as well as an concomitant increase in ICP).

♦ Nondepolarizing neuromuscular blockers must be used with great caution—if at all—in patients with neuromuscular pathology

♦ Depolarizing neuromuscular blockade (i.e., succinylcholine) will increase intracranial, intraocular, and intragastric pressures

Table 5
Properties of Selected Paralytics (Neuromuscular Blockers) in the Neuro-ICU

Drug	Mechanism of action	Advantages	Disadvantages	Metabolism
Succinylcholine (Anectine)	Depolarizing neuromuscular blocker	Rapid onset and elimination	Increased intracranial, intraocular, and intragastric pressures Risk of hyperkalemia; malignant hyperthermia in susceptible patients	Plasma cholinesterase (pseudocholinesterase)
Pancuronium (Pavulon)	Nondepolarizing neuromuscular blocker (competitive nicotinic antagonist)	Longer duration = less intermittent dosing, no effect on ICP, reversible	Tachycardia, prolonged duration in renal impairment; rare histamine release	Renal
Vecuronium (Norcuron)	Nondepolarizing neuromuscular blocker (competitive nicotinic antagonist)	Shorter duration = easily titrated, no effect on ICP, reversible	Duration somewhat unpredictable	Hepatic
Rocuronium (Zemuron)	Nondepolarizing neuromuscular blocker (competitive nicotinic antagonist)	Rapid onset, shorter duration = easily titrated, no effect on ICP, reversible	Cost	Hepatic

Table 6
Administration of Selected Paralytics (Neuromuscular Blockers) in the Neuro-ICU

Drug	Starting dose	Increase by	Maximum dose	Duration of action
Succinylcholine (Anectine)	0.3–1.1 mg/kg bolus	Infusion: 2.5–4.3 mg/min, intermittent: bolus 0.04–0.07 mg/kg	Variable, but generally <10 mg/min	4–6 min (prolonged with pseudocholinesterase deficiency).
Pancuronium (Pavulon)	0.06–0.1 mg/kg bolus	Repeat 0.01 mg/kg based on "train of four" monitoring	Variable	20–60 min (prolonged in renal impairment).
Vecuronium (Norcuron)	0.08–0.1 mg/kg bolus	Infusion: 0.8–1.2 mcg/kg/min, Intermittent: bolus 0.01–0.015 mg/kg based on "train of four" monitoring	Variable	15–45 min (prolonged in hepatic impairment), active metabolites.
Rocuronium (Zemuron)	0.6–1.0 mg/kg bolus	Infusion: 4–16 mcg/kg/min, Intermittent: bolus 0.1–0.15 mg/kg based on "train of four" monitoring	Variable	15–60 min (dose-dependent). Possibly prolonged in hepatic impairment

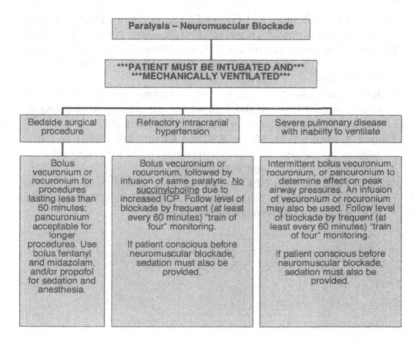

Fig. 3. Flow chart for paralysis in the Neuro-ICU.

Suggested Reading

Miller RD, ed. *Anesthesia,* 5th edition. Philadelphia: Churchill Livingstone; 2000.

Buczko GB. Sedation in critically ill patients: a review. *Med Health RI* 2001;84:321–323.

Hardman JG, and Limbird LE, eds. *Goodman and Gilman's The Pharmacological Basis of Therapeutics,* 10th edition. New York: McGraw-Hill; 2001.

Hemstreet, MK, Suarez, JI, and Mirski, MA. Sedation and analgesia in the critically ill neurology and neurosurgery patient. In: *Critical Care Neurology and Neurosurgery* (Suarez JI, ed.), Totowa, NJ: Humana; 2004:221–245.

Kang TM. Propofol infusion syndrome in critically ill patients. *Ann Pharmacother* 2002;36:1453–1456.

Kelly DF, Goodale DB, Williams J, et al. Propofol in the treatment of moderate and severe head injury: a randomized, prospective double-blinded pilot trial. *J Neurosurg* 1999;90:1042–1052.

Mirski MA, Muffelman B, Ulatowski JA, and Hanley DF. Sedation for the critically ill neurologic patient. *Crit Care Med* 1995;23:2038–2053.

Prasad A, Worrall BB, Bertram EH, and Bleck TP. Propofol and midazolam in the treatment of refractory status epilepticus. *Epilepsia* 2001; 42:380–386.

Sanchez-Izquierdo-Riera JA, Caballero-Cubedo RE, Perez-Vela JL, et al. Propofol versus midazolam: safety and efficacy for sedating the severe trauma patient. *Anesth Analg* 1998;86:1219–1224.

Tipps LB, Coplin WM, Murry KR, and Rhoney DH. Safety and feasibility of continuous infusion of remifentanil in the neurosurgical intensive care unit. *Neurosurgery* 2000;46:596–602.

Venn RM and Grounds RM. Comparison between dexmedetomidine and propofol for sedation in the intensive care unit: patient and clinician perceptions. *Br J Anaesth* 2001;87:684–690.

19 Neurologic Monitoring in the Intensive Care Unit

Connie L. Chen

Situations Requiring Neurologic Monitoring in the Intensive Care Unit and Recommended Monitoring Protocol

♦ Suspicion of elevated intracranial pressure (e.g., tumor, intracranial hemorrhage [ICH], stroke):
- Glasgow Coma Scale (GCS) > 8 and cooperative with exams:
  - Follow neurologic (NRO) exam q h,
  - Diminish NRO checks if stable for 24h (q2h)
  - Head computerized tomography (CT) when patient is stable
- GCS > 8 and uncooperative or difficulty with exams:
  - Follow NRO exam q h
  - Consider ICP monitor
  - Head CT when patient is stable
- GCS ≤ 8 and cooperative with exams:
  - Follow NRO exam q h
  - Consider ICP monitor
  - Head CT when patient is stable
- GCS ≤ 8 and uncooperative or difficulty with exams:
  - Follow NRO exam q h
  - Place ICP monitor
  - Head CT when patient is stable
♦ Aneurysmal subarachnoid hemorrhage (SAH):
- Intact and stable (d 1–3 post aneurysmal rupture):
  - Obtain transcranial Doppler (TCD), establish baseline
- Intact and stable (d 4–14 post aneurysmal rupture):
  - TCD every other day (QOD) while in ICU

From: *Current Clinical Neurology: Handbook of Neurocritical Care*
Edited by: A. Bhardwaj, M. A. Mirski, and J. A. Ulatowski © Humana Press Inc., Totowa, NJ

- Intact and fluctuating neurological exam (d 1–3 post aneurysmal rupture):
  - Obtain TCD, establish baseline
- Intact and fluctuating neurological exam (d 4–14 post aneurysmal rupture):
  - TCD QD
  - Consider cerebral angiogram if severe vasospasm detected by TCDs
- Impaired but stable neurological exam (d 1–3 post aneurysmal rupture):
  - Obtain TCD, establish baseline
  - Head CT when patient is stable
- Impaired but stable neurological exam (d 4–14 post aneurysmal rupture):
  - TCD QD. Consider switching to QOD if still stable by d 7
  - Head CT when patient is stable
- Impaired but fluctuating neurological exam (d 1–3 post aneurysmal rupture):
  - Obtain TCD, establish baseline
  - Head CT when patient is stable
- Impaired but fluctuating neurological exam (d 4–14 post aneurysmal rupture):
  - TCD QD
  - Consider cerebral angiogram for severe vasospasm by TCD
  - Head CT when patient is stable
♦ Seizures and status epilepticus:
  - Single seizure, returned to baseline mental status (MS):
    - Routine electroencephalogram (EEG) for seizure work-up
  - Single seizure, not returned to baseline mental status:
    - Stat EEG for evaluation of status epilepticus
  - Multiple seizures, returned to baseline mental status:
    - Routine EEG for seizure work-up
  - Multiple seizures, not returned to baseline mental status:
    - Stat EEG for evaluation of status epilepticus
  - Status epilepticus:
    - Stat EEG to confirm diagnosis and for continuous EEG monitoring for treatment (identification of burst suppression)
♦ Traumatic brain injury (TBI):
  - GCS > 8:
    - NRO exam, head CT

- GCS ≤ 8
  - NRO exam, head CT
  - Place ICP monitor if abnormal head CT, or if two of the following present:
    - □ Age >40 yr
    - □ Unilateral or bilateral posturing
    - □ Systolic blood pressure (SBP) < 90 mmHg
  - Consider placing jugular bulb catheter to guide therapy
♦ Acute stroke:
  - Monitoring at presentation if time of onset <3h:
    - NRO exam
    - Head CT
  - Monitoring after presentation if time of onset <3h:
    - Patients receiving iv tPA:
      - □ NRO exam q1h × 24h
      - □ Head CT in 24h s/p tPA
    - If no iv tPA is given:
      - □ NRO exam q1–4h
    - Neuroimaging as per stroke work-up
  - Monitoring at presentation if time of onset 3–6h (or 3–12 h in posterior circulation strokes):
    - NRO exam
    - Head CT
    - Consider magnetic resonance imagining/angiography (MRI/A) (with diffusion/perfusion)
    - TCD's for possible
    - Intraarterial (IA) tPA at appropriate medical centers
  - Monitoring after presentation if time of onset 3–6 h (or 3–12 h in posterior circulation strokes):
    - In patients following IA tPA:
      - □ NRO exam q1 h × 24 h
      - □ Head CT in 24h s/p tPA
    - If no IA tPA is given
    - NRO exam q1–4 h
    - Neuroimaging as per stroke work-up
  - Monitoring at presentation if time of onset > 6h (or >12h in posterior circulation strokes):
    - NRO exam
    - Head CT

- Monitoring at presentation if time of onset > 6h (or >12h in posterior circulation strokes):
  - NRO exam q2–4 h
  - Neuroimaging as per stroke work-up

Monitors: Advantages and Limitations

♦ ICP Monitors:
- Subarachnoid bolt:
  - Advantages:
    - □ Low infection risk (<5%)
    - □ May be placed any place on skull
  - Limitations: inaccuracies with:
    - □ High ICP
    - □ Underlying blood clot
    - □ Pressure gradient between left/right supratentorial, or infratentorial compartments
- Intraventricular Catheter (IVC):
  - Advantages:
    - □ Gold standard, considered most accurate in ICP reading
    - □ Only ICP monitor that affords therapeutic option of cerebrospinal fluid (CSF) drainage
  - Limitations:
    - □ Inability of placement with small ventricles
    - □ Infection risk high after 5 d (up to 27%)
    - □ Infection risk increases with irrigation, fluid removal of the drainage system
    - □ Inaccurate when clot, debris, air present in system
    - □ Consider prophylactic treatment with Gram-positive antibiotic coverage
    - □ Consider removing IVC as soon as possible, or changing IVC at 7 d if long-term CSF drainage is required
- Intraparenchymal monitor:
  - Advantages:
    - □ Can directly measure parenchymal pressure
    - □ Does not rely on fluid coupling system (like IVC) for measurements
  - Limitations:
    - □ Infection varies in literature(0–4.4%), but appears less than IVCs
    - □ Readings "drift" substantially after 3 d

- ◆ Transcranial doppler:
  - − Monitoring for vasospasm:
    - • Advantages:
      - □ Noninvasive
      - □ Provides early detection
    - • Limitations:
      - □ Operator dependent (Interobserver variability of approx 10%)
      - □ Patient dependent (lack of acoustic window: black > caucasian patients, female < male, or old > young age)
      - □ Cerebral blood flow varies with gender, hematocrit, age, metabolic perturbations (e.g., hyper- or hypocapnea, temperature)
  - − Intracranial stenosis:
    - • Advantages:
      - □ Provides data in patients unable to have computerized tomography angiography (CTA) or MRA
  - − Emboli detection:
    - • Advantages:
      - □ Can detect asymptomatic emboli and track from one vessel to the next
  - − Collateral cerebral blood flow:
    - • Advantages:
      - □ Can visualize if blood flow is antegrade or retrograde
  - − Sickle cell anemia:
    - • Advantages:
      - □ Treatment dependent on detection of high-velocity state
- ◆ Jugular bulb catheter:
  - − TBI:
    - • Advantages:
      - □ Helps guide therapy to prevent secondary brain injury (SjvO2 < 50% associated with increased mortality.)
      - □ Measures oxygen use from brain tissue (use as indicator of hypoxia)
    - • Limitations:
      - □ Jugular bulbs are not symmetrical in venous drainage from brain. Catheter should be placed on side of higher ICP
      - □ Complications may occur with line placement: pneumothorax, carotid artery puncture, hematoma, thrombus, increased ICP

□ Data does not distinguish between supply and demand

□ Not a quantitative measure. Trending device only

◆ EEG:

   – Seizure ΔMS:

     • Advantages:

        □ Evaluates for seizure or seizure focus

        □ Helps guide therapy for status epilepticus

        □ Can also detect areas of cortical injury secondary to hypoxic, ischemic, or metabolic insult (slowing)

     • Limitations:

        □ Requires ability to read EEG

        □ Sensitive to medications and anesthetics

        □ ICU electrical interference may be a problem

        □ Continuous EEG may be optimal in certain circumstances

        □ Access to bare scalp required

◆ Evoked potentials (somatosensory [SSEP], motor, brainstem auditory [BAEP]):

   – Indications: Brain stem injury, spinal cord injury, and intraoperative monitoring during neurosurgery:

     • Advantages:

        □ Evaluates intactness of sensory or motor pathways from peripheral to cortex

        □ BAEP offer more sensitive indicator of brainstem compromise

        □ May reveal injury during surgery through signal loss

     • Limitations:

        □ Requires skilled technician

        □ Lack of finding does not reflect possible areas of injury outside sensory pathways

        □ Signal quality impaired by interference (cautery)

        □ Sensitive to anesthetics

◆ Electromyography and nerve conduction Studies:

   – Indication: Neuromuscular weakness:

     • Advantages:

        □ Helps differentiate levels of weakness: Muscle vs nerve vs radicular

     • Limitations:

        □ May be inconclusive or not reveal abnormalities in the acute patient.

        □ Operator dependent

Key Points

♦ Neurological exam is invaluable and irreplaceable in early detection of neurologic decline

♦ ICP monitors should be placed in patients who meet head-trauma criteria, have ongoing elevated ICP issues, or have diminished and unreliable exams where ICP may be a concern

♦ Invasive neurologic monitoring may have complications (e.g., infection, bleeding)

Suggested Reading

Bulger EM, Jurkovich, et al. Management of severe head injury: institutional variations in care and effect on outcome. *Crit Care Med* 2002; 30:1870–1806.

Gopinath SP, Robertson CS, et al. Comparison of jugular venous oxygen saturation and brain tissue PO2 as monitors of cerebral ischemia after head injury. *Crit Care Med* 1999;27(11):2337–2345.

Khan, SH, Onyiuke, HC, et al. Comparison of percutaneous ventriculostomies and intraparenchymal monitor: a retrospective evaluation of 156 patients. *Acta Neuro. Suppl* 1998;71:50–52.

Macmillan CSA and Andrews PJD. Cerebrovenous oxygen saturation monitoring: practical considerations and clinical relevance. *Int Care Med* 2000;26:1028–1036.

Markus HS. Transcranial doppler ultrasound. *Brit Med Bull* 2000;56(2): 378–388.

Minahan RE, Bhardwaj A, and Williams MA. Critical Care Monitoring for Cerebralvascualr Disease. *New Horizons* 1997;5(4):406–421.

Piper I, Dunn L, et al. The Camino intracranial pressure sensor: is it optimal technology? An internal audit with a review of current intracranial pressure monitoring technologies. *Neurosurgery* 2001;49(5): 1158–1164.

Robertson CS, Grossman RG, et al. Prevention of secondary insults after sever head injury. *Crit Care Med* 1999;27:2086–2095.

Schell RM and Cole DJ. Cerebral monitoring: jugular venous oximetry. *Anesthesia Analgesia* 2000;90:559–566.

Williams MA and Hanley DF. Monitoring and interpreting intracranial pressure. In: (Tobin MJ, ed.), *Principles and Practice of Intensive Care Monitoring.* New York: McGraw–Hill;1997.

20 Nutrition

Wendy L. Wright

Nutritional Consequences of Critical Illness

♦ Stress of critical illness induces a state of hypermetabolism resulting in a rapid loss of lean body mass, that can lead to increased morbidity and mortality

♦ Malnutrition states are characterized by weight loss, immunosuppression, and poor wound healing

♦ Severe head injury is characterized by negative nitrogen balance,
weight loss, immune depression, and depressed plasma protein level,
even when patients seem to be adequately fed:

– The mechanisms for this state are unclear

♦ Patients often require nonoral nutritional support as a result of
intubation, altered mental status or dysphagia

♦ Early nutritional support has been shown to blunt hypermetabolism, reduce complications, and reduce length of stay

Estimation of Premorbid Nutritional Status

♦ History and physical, looking for signs of malnourishment or
obesity:

– Food intake:

  • Evidence of malabsorption

  • Specific nutrient deficiencies

  • Level of metabolic stress

  • Functional status

♦ Physical examination:

– Tissue depletion

– Muscle function

– Fluid status

– Body weight

From: *Current Clinical Neurology: Handbook of Neurocritical Care*
Edited by: A. Bhardwaj, M. A. Mirski, and J. A. Ulatowski © Humana Press Inc., Totowa, NJ

- Weight is not always reliable given fluid shifts
- Ideal body weight:
  - □ Male: 47.7 kg for the first 5 ft plus 2.7 kg for each inch above 5 ft
  - □ Female: 45 kg for the first 5 ft plus 2.25 kg for each inch above 5 ft
  - □ >200% of ideal body weight: morbidly obese
  - □ 126–199%: obese
  - □ 111–125%: overweight
  - □ 90–110%: adequate energy reserve
  - □ 80–89%: lean body habitus or mildly depleted energy stores
  - □ 70–79%: moderate depletion of energy reserve
  - □ <69%: severe depletion of energy reserve
- Body mass index (BMI):
  - □ Defined as (weight in kg) divided by (height in meters)^2
  - □ Patients can be classified based on BMI as:
    - ◊ <18.5 kg/m^2: underweight
    - ◊ 18.5–24.9 kg/m^2: normal weight
    - ◊ 25.0–29.9 kg/m^2: overweight
    - ◊ 30.0–34.9 kg/m^2: class I obesity
    - ◊ 35.0–39.9 kg/m^2: class II obesity
    - ◊ >40.0 kg/m^2: class III obesity

♦ Energy stores:
  - Calories are derived from the breakdown of carbohydrates, proteins, and fats into their basic constituents and can be converted into:
    - Glucose for immediate energy
    - Glycogen for short-term storage of calories
    - Fat in the form of adipose tissue for long-term storage of calories

♦ Energy expenditure:
  - The ideal way to measure energy requirements is unknown
  - Basal energy expenditure (BEE): heat production of basal metabolism in the resting and fasted state
  - Predictive Equations:
    - Harris–Benedict Equation:
      - □ BEE(kcal/d):
        - ◊ Males: $66 + (13.7 \times wt) + (5 \times ht) - (6.7 \times A)$
        - ◊ Females: $65.5 + (9.6 \times wt) + (1.8 \times ht) - (4.7 \times A)$ where wt is weight in kg, ht is height in cm, and A is age in years

◊ Takes into account the effect of body size and lean tissue mass (which is influenced by body size)
◊ Use current body weight
◊ In the very obese patient use 120 kg because equations are less accurate over this weight
□ Simplified equation:
◊ BEE (kcal/d) = 25–35 × wt (in kg)
◊ Wt is ideal body weight
- Once the BEE is estimated, adjustments can be made to account for extra energy required because of disease state:
  • Fever: BEE × 1.1 (for each °C above the normal body temperature)
  • Minor surgery without complications: BEE × 1.1
  • Mild stress: BEE × 1.2
  • Infection, major surgery without complications: BEE × 1.2
  • Fracture: BEE × 1.35
  • Moderate stress: BEE × 1.4
  • <20% total body surface area burn, multiple fractures: 1.5
  • Severe stress: BEE × 1.6
  • Sepsis, multi-system organ failure, acute respiratory distress syndrome (ARDS), closed head injury: BEE × 1.6–1.8
  • >20% total body surface area burns: BEE × 1.8–2.0
  • BEE is increased on an average of 40% for 3 wk after head injury
  • In spinal cord injury, the BEE is 10–55% lower than predicted
  • In stroke patients, about 20% increase in energy demand, probably caused by increased catecholamines
- Stress stratification estimate:
  • 26 kcal/kg/d after craniotomy
  • 40 to 50 kcal/kg/d for patients with GCS of 4 to 5
  • 30 to 40 kcal/kg/d for patients with GCS of 6 to 7
  • 30 to 35 kcal/kg.d for patients with GCS of 8 to 12
  • 27 kcal/kg/d for paraplegic patients
  • 23 kcal/kg/d for quadriplegic patients
  • 6 to 10 kcal/kg/d for patients with brain death
  • 60 kcal/kg/d for patients in status epilepticus
  • 15 to 18 kcal/kg/d for patients in barbiturate coma
- Resting energy expenditure (REE): Energy expenditure of the basal metabolism in the resting but not fasted state:
  • Indirect calorimetry:

- □ An instrument called a metabolic cart measures the exchange of O_2 and CO_2 across the lungs for 15–30 min and this is extrapolated over 24 h
- REE and respiratory quotient (RQ) by metabolic cart:
  - □ REE (kcal/24 h) = $(3.9 \times VO_2) + (1.1 \times VCO_2) - 61$
    - ◊ This equation is not reliable if $FIO_2 > 50\%$ or positive end-expiratory pressure (PEEP) >10
- The Fick equation can be used to calculate energy expenditure in patients who have a pulmonary artery catheter in place:
  - REE (kcal/d) = $(SaO_2 - SvO_2) \times CO \times Hb \times 95.18$
  Where SaO_2 and SvO_2 are the percent oxygen saturation in arterial and mixed venous blood (in fractions), respectively; CO is cardiac output (in L/min); and Hb is hemoglobin (in g/dL)
- ♦ Once caloric requirements are estimated, the requirements of protein, carbohydrate and fat must be determined:
  - Protein requirements:
    - 15–25% total kcal
    - Protein has 4 kcal/g
    - In normal metabolism: 0.6–1.0 grams of protein/kg of body weight/d
    - In critical illness/hypermetabolism: 1.2–1.6 g/kg/d
    - In head injury: 1.5 to 2.5 g/kg/d
    - Renal failure:
      - □ No stress, no dialysis 0.6–0.8
      - □ Metabolic stress, no dialysis 0.8–1.0 d/kg/d
      - □ Hemodialysis 1.2–1.4 g/kg/d
      - □ Peritoneal dialysis 1.2–1.5 g/kg/d
      - □ Continuous veno-venous hemofiltration (CVVHD)/continuous arterio-venous hemodialysis (CAVHD) 1.5–1.8g/kg/d
  - Carbohydrate requirements:
    - Dextrose has 3.4 kcal/g; sucrose has 4 kcal/g
    - The brain prefers glucose as a fuel
    - Peripheral nerves, eye tissues, bone marrow, erythrocytes, leukocytes, and the renal medulla can not metabolize fatty acids and require glucose as a fuel
    - Avoid excessive intake of carbohydrates
      - □ Carbohydrates stimulate the release of insulin that inhibits the mobilization of free fatty acids from adipose tissue, thus limiting the body's ability to rely on endogenous fat stores

    □ Can be accompanied by excessive CO_2 production, promoting hypercapnia if lung function is compromised
- Lipid requirements:
  - Fat has 9 kcal /g
  - 30–40% of calories should be provided by fat starting with a carbohydrate:lipid ratio of 4:1
  - Increase lipid and decrease carbohydrates if hyperglycemic or insulin-resistant
  - Minimal 10% of kcal to prevent essential fatty acid deficiency (EFAD), linoleic acid and linolenic acid:
    - □ EFAD: scaly dermopathy, immunosuppression, hemolytic anemia, increased platelet aggregation, cardiac dysfunction, decreased wound healing and hepatic dysfunction
  - Maximum 60% total kcal or 2 g/kg of body weight
    - □ Avoid providing more than 50–60% of calories from lipid
    - □ Fat overload syndrome: fatty deposition in capillary beds of major organs, resulting in organ failure, thrombocytopenia, and hemolytic anemia
  - Reduce amount of lipids administered if triglycerides >300
  - Note that Propofol is 10% lipid-based and frequently used for ICU sedation
- Micronutrients: important for ionic equilibrium, water balance, and function of enzyme complexes:
  - Major minerals
  - Essential vitamins
  - Essential trace elements
- ◆ Fluid requirements:
  - The goal, in most patients, is euvolemia
  - By weight: 25–35mL/kg per day depending on age, sex, activity
  - By calories: 1mL of fluid/kcal of nutrient intake
  - Limit in congestive heart failure (CHF), oliguria, hyponatremia, syndrome of inappropriate secretion of antidiuretic hormone (SIADH)
  - Increase if abnormal gastrointestinal (GI), skin or renal fluid losses
  - Consider all sources of fluid: IV, enteral, oral, medications
  - Fluid balance should by monitored daily, and insensible losses of 500 mL/d, plus 300 mL/d/°C in a febrile patient, should be accounted for

- Fluids given to replenish volume losses should not be hypotonic

Nutritional Monitoring

♦ It is impossible to determine the exact daily energy requirements by using predictive equations because of the complexity of factors that affect metabolic rate. Therefore the calculated energy requirements should be modified as needed based on the patient's clinical course
♦ Laboratory tests are essential in following the effectiveness of nutritional therapy, and in diagnosing specific nutrient deficiencies:
    – Check electrolytes daily when nutritional therapy is initiated, and 3–5 times a week when a relatively stable nutritional regimen is achieved
♦ Assess protein stores:
    – Support of visceral protein synthesis as judged by acute-phase reactant and hepatic protein synthesis
    – Measurement of protein stores may be unreliable if creatinine clearance is under 50 mL/min or if patients in are in fulminant renal or hepatic failure:
    • Albumin:
        □ Adequate: 3.5–5.0 mg/dL
        □ Mildly depleted: 2.8–3.4 mg/dL
        □ Moderately depleted: 2.1–2.7 mg/dL
        □ Severely depleted: <2.1 mg/dL
        □ Serum albumin measurement is unreliable after fluid resuscitation has begun and the acute stress response has occurred
    • Transferrin:
        □ Adequate: 212–360 mg/dL
        □ Mildly depleted:150–211 mg/dL
        □ Moderately depleted: 100–149 mg/dL
        □ Severely depleted: <100 mg/dL
    • Prealbumin:
        □ Adequate: 18–45 mg/dL
        □ Mildly depleted: 15–17 mg/dL
        □ Moderately depleted: 11–14 mg/dL
        □ Severely depleted: <10 mg/dL
        □ Prealbumin is the most sensitive measure and often the test of choice

♦ Nitrogen Balance:
  - Urine collected for 24 h and total urine urea nitrogen (UUN) is determined:
  - Nitrogen balance = (protein intake/6.25 [g/d]) – (Urine nitrogen/0.8[g/d] + GI losses [2–4 g/d] + cutaneous loss [0–4 g/d])
  - Approximation of nitrogen balance:
  N balance (g) = (Protein intake (g)/6.25) – (UUN + 4)
  Where UUN is the urinary urea nitrogen excretion in grams over 24 h
  - The goal of nutritional repletion is a positive nitrogen balance of 4–6 g
  - Provide enough nonprotein calories to spare proteins from being degraded to provide energy:
    • If the protein intake is constant, nitrogen balance becomes positive only when the intake of nonprotein calories is sufficient to meet the daily energy needs
    • If the nonprotein calories are insufficient, some of the protein provided in the diet will be broken down for calories and that will produce a negative nitrogen balance
    • Therefore, if the daily intake of nonprotein calories is insufficient, increasing the protein intake becomes an inefficient method of achieving nitrogen balance
  - Metabolic cart:
    • The respiratory quotient (RQ) is calculated as the ratio of VCO_2 to VO_2 and used with the 24-h UUN to calculate the source of energy predominantly used by the patient, if desired
    • RQ = $(3.586 \times VO_2) + (1.433 \times VCO_2) - 1.180$ NM
    • NM is metabolized nitrogen (grams of protein intake/6.25)
    • RQ = 0.7 indicates predominant fat usage, RQ = 0.8 protein and RQ = 1.0 carbohydrate; RQ > 1 may indicate overfeeding
    • RQ can be estimated using the Fick method with a pulmonary artery catheter, although this is less accurate
  - Nutritional monitoring may help in avoiding complications of excess VCO_2 and urea production, blood urea nitrogen (BUN) less than 110 mg/%

Nutrient Toxicity

♦ Carbohydrate can be used to generate lactic acid, a metabolic toxin, when nutrient processing is abnormal
♦ Complications of overfeeding: Excessive CO_2 production, increased minute ventilation, respiratory failure, respiratory acidosis

in chronic obstructive pulmonary disease (COPD) as a result of CO_2
retention, pulmonary edema, worsening of CHF, hyperglycemia, lipo-
genesis, gain of fluid/fat rather than lean body mass, fatty liver,
uremia, electrolyte depletion
♦ Consequences of overfeeding: life-threatening fluid and electrolyte
shifts (e.g., refeeding syndrome), azotemia, hypertonic dehydration,
metabolic acidosis, hypercapnia, hyperglycemia, hyperlipidemia, and
hepatic steatosis

Oral Feeding

♦ Candidates for oral feeding should be extubated, alert, and able to
follow commands. They should have intact swallowing and adequate
GI function
♦ Oral feeding should not be considered if the patient is unable to
swallow or protect their airway
♦ When in doubt, a bedside swallowing evaluation can be performed
♦ Close observation is necessary when feeding patients with hemiparesis as they may be apraxic and can have neglect of food in their
mouths, thus increasing the risk of aspiration
♦ Oral feeding may be difficult if patients have nausea or vomiting,
intolerable post-prandial abdominal pain, or high-output fistulas
♦ Hospital diets include a regular diet and diets modified in either
nutrient content (e.g., sodium, fat, sugar, protein) or consistency (e.g.,
soft, pureed, liquid); or in order to account for dietary preferences (e.g.,
vegetarian or Kosher meals) or food intolerances (e.g., lactose-free)
♦ Use a calorie count to ensure adequate caloric intake
♦ If caloric intake is inadequate, attempts should be made to:
  – Provide assistance with meals especially in patients with oral
  apraxia or neglect
  – Limit meals missed for medical tests or procedures
  – Avoid unpalatable diets and/or allow some food to be supplied
  by the patient's visitors
  – Encourage PO intake
♦ If the patient deteriorates or is unable to take in adequate nutrition,
enteral or parenteral therapy may be needed

Enteral Therapy

♦ Whenever possible, the gut should be used to provide nutrients in
order to maintain structural and functional integrity of the intestinal
mucosa and the pancreas

♦ Trophism and sepsis:
  – Depletion of the bowel lumen is accompanied by degenerative changes in bowel mucosa
  – Translocation:
    • Enteric pathogens move across the bowel mucosa and into the systemic circulation, likely because of mucosal disruption from lack of luminal nutrients
    • Burn patients are much more susceptible to translocation and enteral feedings should be started as soon as possible
    • Indications for enteral therapy: inadequate nutrient intake for more than five days, intubated patients, patients who are unable to swallow or who are unable to take adequate amounts of calories orally
♦ Contraindications to enteral therapy: circulatory shock, intestinal ischemia, complete mechanical bowel obstruction, ileus, and pharmacologic coma
♦ Feeding a hemodynamically unstable patient may lead to undesirable complications, most notably bowel infarction in enterally fed patients
♦ Total enteral nutrition may not be possible in conditions of severe hypomotility, severe malabsorption, diarrhea, or high-output fistulas. However, low-volume enteric feedings may be tolerated and may help to maintain intestinal integrity
♦ Routes of administration:
  – Short-term (less than 2 wk of tube feeds anticipated)
    • Nasal tube feedings: nasogastric, nasoduodenal, nasojejunal:
      □ May be contraindicated in nasal or facial trauma, or after certain neurosurgical or ENT procedures
      □ May contribute to the development of sinusitis
    • Nasogastric tube:
      □ Standard tubes (14 to 16 French) are often uncomfortable for conscious patients. Soft, narrower (8 to 10 French) tubes are more comfortable, but may limit the delivery of pills:
        ◊ Clinical studies *do not* support the belief that larger tubes promote gastroesophageal reflux
    • Oral tube feedings:
      □ Used more frequently in intubated patients vs extubated patients
      □ May be contraindicated in jaw or facial trauma
    • Checking tube position:
      □ Chest radiograph
      □ Auscultation
      □ Gastric pH

- Long-term (>2 wk) feeding tubes:
  - Surgical or endoscopic tube placement is advantageous over temporary tube placement because:
    - They have a larger diameter and therefore are less likely to clog
    - They are fixed to the stomach or intestines and therefore will not migrate into the esophagus, thereby reducing the risk of aspiration
    - They are more comfortable and often more aesthetically acceptable for the patient
  - Gastrostomy
  - Percutaneous endoscopic gastrostomy (PEG):
    - Has become the most common type of long-term feeding tube placement because of the ease of performing the procedure and the relatively low risk
  - Jejunostomy:
    - Motility of the small bowel is often unimpaired after surgery, and patients can often tolerate feedings into the jejunum within hours of surgery
- The feeding site (gastric feeding vs duodenal feeding vs jejunal feeding):
  - A pilot study of critically ill neurologic patients showed no increased risk or benefit of gastric vs duodenal feeding
  - Brain-injured patients may exhibit altered gastric emptying. Thus, some believe post-pyloric feeding to be tolerated better than gastric feeding
  - However, reliable post-pyloric access can be difficult to obtain, so gastric feeding remains the preferred route for administering nutrition
- Tube feed administration:
  - Tube feeds are often started at a low rate and advanced as tolerated:
  - Starter regimen:
    - Traditionally, tube feeds were started with dilute formulas and at a slow infusion rate and gradually advanced.This presumably gives the atrophic bowel mucosa time to regenerate after a period of bowel rest
    - Starter regimens are *not* necessary for gastric feedings
    - Starter regimens may be required for duodenal and jejunal feedings

- Gastric retention:
  - If residuals are more than 150 cc, hold tube feeds for 2 h
  - Promotility agents such as metoclopramide or erythromycin may reduce gastric residuals
  - If residuals remain high, duodenal or jejunal feedings may be necessary
  - Bowel sounds are an unreliable indicator or small bowel function
  - Studies indicate patients with severe neurologic deficits and clinically silent abdomens can tolerate low-rate jejunal feedings within 36 h of injury or surgery and can increase rate to meet goals within 2–4 d
  - If tube feeds are started prior to pentobarbital infusion, even patients in pentobarbital coma can often be fed enterally
- Feeding schedule:
  - Continuous gastric feeding is better tolerated than bolus feedings in patients with acute brain injuries, likely because of delayed gastric emptying
    - □ Can usually be started at a rate of 20–40 mL per hour and advanced as rapidly as 10 cc per hour until the goal rate
    - □ Patients with gastroparesis may need to be started on a rate of 10mL/h and advanced by 10mL every 8–12 h
    - □ Infused for 12–16 h/d
    - □ Continuous infusion without bowel rest is an unrelenting stress to the bowel mucosa and promotes malabsorption and diarrhea
    - □ Continuous feeding should always be used for duodenal or jejunal feeds
  - Intermittent bolus feeding more closely approximates the normal condition, but the volumes required are often too large to be tolerated or given safely
    - □ Determine the total amount of daily formula and divide it into four to six equal portions
    - □ The patient's upper body should be elevated by 30–45 (during and for at least 2 h after feeding)
- ◆ Formulation of tube feeds:
  - Over 80 enteral feeding formulas are available
  - Caloric density:
    - Standard caloric density formulas provide 1–1.5 kcal/L
    - High caloric density formulas provide 1.5–2 kcal/L, which is better for patients who are volume restricted

- Osmolality: Directly related to caloric density, ranges from 280 to 1100 mOsm/kg H_2O
  - Lower caloric density formulas (1 kcal/L) are often isotonic to body fluids (approx 300 mOsm/kg H_2O)
  - Higher caloric density formulas (2 kcal/L) are hypertonic (approx1000 mOsm/kg H_2O)
- Protein content:
  - Standard formulas provide 35–40 g/protein/L
  - Higher protein formulas (often designated HN for "high nitrogen") provide about 20% more protein that standard formulas
  - Protein complexity:
    □ Some formulas contain small peptides instead of intact protein because these peptides are more readily absorbed
  - Can be used in patients with impaired intestinal absorption
  - These formulas promote water re-absorption from the bowel, and therefore may be beneficial in patients with severe diarrhea
- Lipids:
  - Excessive fat ingestion is not well tolerated and promotes diarrhea
  - Lipid rich formulas are intended for patients with respiratory failure
  - Fat complexity:
    □ Alternative lipids
- Additives:
  - Glutamine: the principle fuel for bowel mucosa; supplementation may prevent bowel ischemia
  - Plant fiber:
    □ Fermentable: Slows gastric emptying and binds bile salts that can alleviate diarrhea
    □ Nonfermentable: not degraded by intestinal bacteria, creates an osmotic force that adsorbs water from the bowel lumen, and therefore can reduce watery diarrhea
◆ Classifications of feeding solutions:
- Blenderized foods
  - Natural foods that are semiliquified in a blender
- Polymeric solutions:
  - Solutions containing nitrogen in the form of whole proteins, carbohydrate polymers and intact triglycerides
  - These solutions can be used as oral supplements

- Monomeric solutions:
  - Solutions that contain nitrogen in the form of peptides and/or amino acids, carbohydrates in the form of partially hydrolyzed starch, and fat as a mixture of medium- and long-chain triglycerides
  - Intended for patients with impaired digestion or absorption
  - Not palatable to be given as oral feedings
- Solutions for specific metabolic needs:
  - Designed for patients with hepatic failure, renal failure, respiratory failure, trauma, or inborn errors of metabolism
- Modular solutions:
  - Consist of single nutrients that can be given by themselves or mixed with other enteral formulas to provide special nutritional or metabolic needs
- ◆ Complications:
  - Tube-related complications:
    - Insertion-related complications:
      - □ Trauma and bleeding from the nose and upper GI tract
      - □ Perforation of the GI tract
      - □ Misplacement of the tube:
        - ◊ Particularly into the respiratory tract of unconscious patients
        - ◊ Intracranial placement can occur in patients with skull fractures
        - ◊ Respiratory compromise caused by coiling of the tube in the nasopharynx
      - □ Vomiting of gastric contents as a result of pharyngeal irritation
    - Postinsertion complications:
      - □ Clogging, kinking, or bursting of the tube
        - ◊ Clogging can be reduced by avoiding administration of pill fragments or thick solutions
        - ◊ Bursting can be avoided by not forcefully administering solutions
      - □ Migration of the tube, especially into the esophagus
      - □ Aspiration of infused solutions
      - □ Erosion of the GI tract mucosa by the tip of the tube which can lead to GI tract perforation
      - □ Erosive tissue damage can also lead to nasopharyngeal erosions, pharyngitis, sinusitis, and otitis media

– Metabolic:
  • Patients with renal failure are at risk for developing increased azotemia, hyperkalemia, hypermagnesemia, and hyperphosphatemia
  • Patients with diabetes are at risk for hyperglycemia
  • Dehydration is a potential complication in patients given high-osmolality enteral feeding solutions
– GI complications:
  • Feeding intolerance
    □ Independent predictors of feeding intolerance:
      ◊ Medications: Sucralfate, propofol, pentobarbital, or use of paralytics
      ◊ Older age
      ◊ Days receiving mechanical ventilation
      ◊ Admission diagnosis of either intracerebral hemorrhage or ischemic stroke
  • The frequency of enteral feeding interruptions may indicate inadequate nutritional support
  • Diarrhea:
    □ Diarrhea may develop from tube feeds because of high osmolality
    □ May be alleviated by diluting tube feeds with water, switching to another formula, cutting the rate of feeds, or adding fiber to the tube feeds
    □ Calculate stool osmotic gap = serum osmality – 2 × (stool Na^+ + stool K):
      ◊ A large gap (>100) indicates osmotic diarrhea
        ○ Consider altering fat/fiber/nutrient density of enteral formula if large gap
      ◊ A small (≤100) or negative gap indicates a secretory diarrhea
        ○ Obtain *C. difficile* assay and fecal leukocytes, review medications for potential contributors
    □ If diarrhea persists after adequate evaluation of other possible causes, a trail of antidiarrheal agents, fiber administration, or supplemental lactobacillus acidophilus may be of benefit
  • Constipation:
    □ Rule out other causes of decreased stool output, such as fecal impaction, ileus or obstruction

□ Neuro ICU patients without diarrhea should be on a bowel regimen including daily stool softeners. If stool output is inadequate, a suppository can be given daily or every other day; if the suppository is ineffective, QOD enemas should be administered
- • Nausea and vomiting
- − Infectious complications:
  - • Aspiration pneumonia:
    □ Risk factors for aspiration include misplacement of the tip of the feeding tube in the esophagus or upper stomach, impaired gastric emptying, decreased lower esophageal sphincter pressure, large feeding volume, patient's position during feeding, and various medications that decrease GI peristalsis
    □ Risk of aspiration is equal in gastric and duodenal feedings
    □ In patients with impaired gastric emptying and no gag reflex, jejunal feeding may decrease the aspiration risk
    □ Risk of aspiration can be reduced by appropriately positioning the feeding tube, elevating the upper body to 30–45° and avoiding enteral feeding when contraindicated
    □ It is often impossible to discern if the aspiration was caused by aspirated gastric contents or aspirated oropharyngeal secretions
    □ Coloring tube feeds had been a helpful, but not always reliable, way to diagnose aspiration:
    ◊ However, recent data indicates that blue tube feed dye can be absorbed when administered to critically ill patients, and cause unwanted side effects including metabolic acidosis, hypotension, skin discoloration
    ◊ Many ICUs are abandoning this practice
  - • Sepsis is occasionally reported:
    □ Enteral feeding formulas are an ideal growth medium for bacteria
- ♦ Transition to oral feeding:
  - − When swallow evaluation is successful:
    • Give supplemental tube feeds (continuous at night or bolus after each meal) to provide 50% of calorie and protein needs
    • Advance diet with nutritional supplements per dietician/speech pathologist
    • Have nursing staff assist patient with all meals and supplements

- Monitor oral intake
- Adjust tube feeds per PO intake
- Place back on 24-h tube feeds if intake <70% of goal, declining prealbumin or weight loss
- Discontinue supplemental tube feeds when oral intake >70% of goal, normal prealbumin and weight stable
- If patient is unable to tolerate enteral support or achieve or maintain adequate goal restart total parental nutrition (TPN) or peripheral parental nutrition (PPN)

Parenteral Therapy

♦ Indications
  – Energy intake that has been, or is expected to be, inadequate (< 50% of daily requirements) for more than 7 d
  – When full nutritional support is not possible with enteral tube feedings
  – TPN: indicated in patients with inadequate small bowel function or in whom all forms of enteral access or support are contraindicated and who have central venous access
  – PPN: indicated in patients with inadequate small bowel function or if all forms of enteral access are contraindicated ≤7 d, or all forms of central venous access are contraindicated
  – Routes of delivery—TPN:
    • Large-bore high-flow vessels to minimize irritation and damage with the infusion of hyperosmolar nutrient solution
      □ Percutaneous subclavian vein catheterization with the tip of the catheter at the junction of the superior vena cava with the right atrium
      □ Femoral central line
      □ Internal jugular central line
      □ Peripherally inserted intravenous central catheter (PICC) lines through the antecubital vein
♦ Formulations:
  – Macronutrient solutions:
    • Crystalline amino acid solutions
    • Glucose
    • Lipid emulsions
  – Additives:
    • Electolytes: sodium, chloride, potassium, magnesium, calcium, and phosphorous can all be added to TPN to replace normal daily electrolyte losses

- Vitamins: an aqueous multivitamin preparation can be added to the dextrose-amino acid mixtures, and this will provide the normal daily requirements for most vitamins, except for vitamin K
  - Some vitamins are degraded before delivery, and may need additional supplementation
  - Vitamin A is degraded by light
  - Thiamine is degraded by sulfite ions used as preservatives for amino acid solutions
- Trace elements: most trace element mixtures contain chromium, copper, manganese, and zinc, but not iron or iodine; some mixtures contain selenium
- Glutamine

♦ TPN administration:
  - Obtain fresh central venous access and administer TPN through a clean, dedicated port
  - The goal of TPN is to provide 100% of calorie/protein/micronutrient needs
  - Standard TPN contains 50 g of protein and 850 nonprotein kcal/L
  - Nonstandard TPN: for patients with diabetes, insulin resistance, renal or hepatic dysfunction, refeeding syndrome risk, fluid restriction, electrolyte abnormalities
  - Formulation is best done with the aid of a nutritional consult:
    - Estimate the daily calorie and protein requirements. For example:
      - Calorie requirement = 25(kcal/kg) × wt (in kg)
      - Protein requirement = 1.4(g/d) × wt (in kg)
      - Determine the volume of TPN mixture required to deliver the estimated daily protein requirement
      - For standard 10% amino acids (500 mL) and 50% dextrose (500 mL) mixture, there are 50 g/protein/L, so divide the protein requirements in g/d by 50 g/L to get the volume in L/d
      - Divide this by 24 h to get a per-hour infusion rate
      - Determine the total calories that will be provided by the dextrose in the mixture
      - Multiply the amount of dextrose in g/L by the amount of solution in L/d to get g/d, then multiplying by 3.4 kcal/g
    - Add 10% lipid emulsion (1 kcal/mL) in an amount sufficient to provide for the remaining calories required (e.g., lipid solutions are often infused twice a week)

□ Intralipid solutions: 10% contains 1.1 kcal/cc, 20% contains 2 kcal/cc

□ Patients with hypertriglyceridemia (>300 mg%) or pancreatitis caused by hyperlipidemia should not receive lipid infusions

• Add standard electrolytes, vitamins, and trace elements
• Add insulin as needed
• Monitor electrolytes, triglycerides, and glucose levels daily

– If nutritional requirements are met as soon as possible, the ICU stays are shorter and infectious complications are less

– Give a small rate of tube feeds into the gut if possible to preserve GI mucosa, while decreasing the amount of TPN as enteral feeds are advanced

♦ PPN administration:

– Parental nutrition can occasionally be delivered via peripheral veins for short periods of time (several days)

– Osmolarity should be kept below 900 mOSM/L to prevent osmotic damage to the vessels, and must therefore be delivered with dilute amino acid and dextrose solution

– Because lipid emulsions are isotonic to plasma, lipids can be used to provide a significant amount of the nonprotein calories in PPN

– The goal of PPN is to provide just enough nonprotein calories to spare the breakdown of proteins to provide energy

• <10% amino acid solution
• <20 initial/12.5% final dextrose concentration
• <2 grams lipid/kg/d, NTE 60% of total kcal

– Minimize additives to reduce osmolality:

• Vitamins, insulin, H2 blockers, and standard electrolytes can generally be added to solution if no other access route is available

– Assess appropriateness or peripheral parenteral support and patient's ability to tolerate it

• Patient should meet four criteria for standard PPN
  □ Serum triglycerides <200
  □ Good peripheral IV access
  □ Able to tolerate three liters of IV volume daily
  □ All forms of enteral feeding and central venous access contraindicated

– If the patient does not meet all four criteria, reconsider enteral feeds or start nutritional support via central line

♦ Complications of parenteral nutrition:
  – Catheter related:
    • Pneumothorax
    • Misdirected catheter
    • Thrombosis and pulmonary embolism
  – Metabolic:
    • Metabolic bone disease
    • Carbohydrate complications:
      □ Hyperglycemia
        ◊ Can sometimes be reduced by limiting the non-protein calories provided by dextrose in favor of adding lipids
        ◊ However, persistent hyperglycemia often requires the addition of insulin to TPN solutions
        ◊ Patients will require more insulin if added to TPN than if delivered otherwise because insulin adsorbs to all plastics and glass used in the infusion sets
        ◊ The insulin dose can be adjusted to achieve the desired glycemic control
  – Carbon dioxide retention:
    • Attributed to carbohydrate overfeeding and the high respiratory quotient associated with carbohydrate metabolism, but may be a reflection of overfeeding in general
    • Hypophosphatemia:
      □ A result of enhanced uptake of phosphate into cells associated with glucose entry into cells
  – GI complications:
    • Bowel atrophy: glutamine-supplemented TPN may help reduce this complication
    • Acalculous cholecystitis: caused by the absence of lipids in the proximal small bowel
    • Hepatobilliary complications:
      □ Fatty liver:
        ◊ When glucose requirements exceed the daily calorie requirement, lipogenesis in the liver can progress to fatty infiltration of the liver and blood transaminase levels can increase
        ◊ It is unclear whether or not this process has any pathologic consequences
  – Infectious complications:
    • Catheter-related sepsis

- Complications of lipid infusion:
  - Oxidation-induced cell injury
  - Impaired oxygenation
  - Hyperlipidemia
  - Electrolyte abnormalities
- Special Issues:
  - Re-feeding syndrome
    - Risk when feeding malnourished patients:
      ◊ Significant intracellular shifts of potassium, magnesium, phosphate and fluids leading to hypokalemia, hypomagnesemia, and hypophosphotemia
      ◊ Increased risk of significant morbidity and mortality
      ◊ Best prevented by regular assessment and repletion of electrolytes
- ◆ Stress Ulcers:
  - Risk factors:
    - Respiratory failure
    - Hypotension
    - Sepsis
    - Coagulopathy
    - Renal failure
    - Hepatic failure
    - Jaundice
    - Peritonitis
    - Burns of >25% body surface area
    - Steroid use
  - Stress ulcer bleeding in patients with head trauma correlates with the severity of injury, regardless of the presence of other risk factors
  - Protective factors:
    - Enteral nutrition: possibly caused by dilutional alkalinization that may occur when tube feeds are delivered into the stomach
    - Adequate nutrition: provides a positive nitrogen balance, which is important for normal reparative functions
  - Stress ulcer prophylaxis:
    - Antacids: elevate pH quickly for a sustained period of time
      - Examples: magnesium hydroxide, aluminum hydroxide or aluminum-magnesium mixtures
      - Side effects: in large doses, these include diarrhea or constipation, electrolyte abnormalities, hypophosphatemia (secondary to their phosphate-binding properties), and metabolic alkalosis

□ Primary route of excretion for magnesium and aluminum may also be compromised in renal failure

• Histamine receptor antagonists: reversible inhibition of parietal cell histamine Type 2 receptors reduces acid secretion:

□ Examples: cimetidine, ranitidine and famotidine.

□ At least as efficacious as antacids

□ Central nervous system (CNS) toxicity with cimetidine (which is no longer available in the United States), occurs in a dose-related fashion in less than 3% of patients. Cimetidine and ranitidine both cross the blood–brain barrier

□ CNS side effects of restlessness, confusion, disorientation, agitation, visual hallucinations, muscular twitching, seizures, unresponsiveness, and apnea

□ Other major side effects of H2 antagonists include the inhibition of the cytochrome P450 enzyme system, interference with antibiotic activity, hypotension, and thrombocytopenia

• Sucralfate:

□ Consists of a complex of sucrose, sulfates, and aluminum hydroxide. Its protective effect is exerted through its mucosal strengthening action

□ Sucralfate binds to normal and defective gastric mucosa, and increases the viscosity and mucin content of the gastric mucosa

□ Some other beneficial effects have been reported including inhibition of peptic digestion, stimulation of prostaglandin, protection of the mucosal proliferative zone, facilitation of mucosal regeneration and healing, and bactericidal properties

□ Sucralfate is at least as effective as antacids, and probably more effective than H2 antagonists

□ Side effects can include aluminum retention in patients with renal failure, decreased bioavailability of a number of drugs if they are not given at least 2 h before sucralfate

• Proton pump inhibitors:

□ Examples: omeprazole, lansoprazole, pantoprazole

□ CNS side effects are uncommon but may include headache or mild dizziness

– Nosocomial pneumonia: there is concern for increased incidence of nosocomial pneumonia with pH-altering stress ulcer prophylaxis, as the high pH in the stomach has an important bactericidal effect

• Comparative studies reveal conflicting results, but it is likely that sulcralfate use has a lower incidence of pneumonia than other therapies

Key Points

♦ Brain-injured patients have higher basal energy expenditure and require increased caloric intake
♦ Brain-injured patients usually have difficulties with required daily intake. Swallow study is recommended when in doubt
♦ Enteral feeding is preferred but gastroparesis occurs commonly in brain-injured patients

Suggested Reading

Day L, Stotts NA, Frankfurt A, et al. Gastric versus duodenal feeding in patients with neurological disease: a pilot study. *J. Neurosci. Nurs.* 2001;33(3):148–149, 155–159.

Kocan MJ and Hickisch SM. A comparison of continuous and intermittent enteral nutrition in NICU patients. *J Neurosci. Nurs.* 1986;18(6): 333–337.

Nataloni S, Gentili P, Marini B, et al. Nutritional assessment in head injured patients through the study of rapid turnover visceral proteins. *Clin. Nutr.* 1999;18(4):247–251.

Negro F and Cerra FB. Nutritional monitoring in the ICU: rational and practical application. *Crit. Care. Clin.* 1988;4(3):559–572.

Rhoney DH, Parker D, Formea CM, et al. Tolerability of bolus versus continuous gastric feeding in brain-injured patients. *Neurol. Res.* 2002; 24:613–620.

Ghanbari C. Protocols for nutrition support of neuro intensive care unit patients: a guide for residents. *Inter. J. Emer. Int. Care. Med.* 1999;3.

Marino PL, ed. *The ICU Book,* 2nd edition, Philadelphia: Lippincott, Williams and Wilkins; 1998:721–736, 737–753, 754–765.

Ott L, Annis K, Hatton J, et al. Post-pyloric enteral feeding costs for patients with severe head injury: blind placement, endoscopy, and PEG/J versus TPN. *J. Neurotrauma.* 1999;16:233–242.

Rapp RP, Young B, Twyman D, et al. The favorable effect of early parenteral feeding on survival in head-injured patients. *J Neurosurg* 1983; 58:906–912.

Shils ME, Olson JE, Shike M, et al. *Modern Nutrition in Health and Disease,* 9th edition. Baltimore: Lippincott, Williams and Wilkins; 1998: 1643–1688.

21 Neuroleptic Malignant Syndrome

Connie L. Chen

Epidemiology

- ♦ Incidence:
  - – 0.07–2.2% of those exposed to neuroleptics
- ♦ Population at risk:
  - – Patients on neuroleptics
  - – Patients with Parkinson's disease
  - – Alcoholics
- ♦ Risk factors:
  - – Previous history of neuroleptic malignant syndrome (NMS)
  - – Exposure to any neuroleptics, including "atypical," or dopamine antagonists
  - – Abrupt withdrawal of dopamine or dopamine agonists
  - – Parenteral or intramuscular administration of neuroleptics
  - – Alcoholism
  - – Dehydration
  - – Agitation
- ♦ Poor prognosticators:
  - – Renal failure:
    - • Female gender*
    - • Older age*
    - *Based on one study
- ♦ Pathogenesis:
  - – Theories include central dopamine receptor blockade and peripheral skeletal muscle susceptibility to dopamine blockade
- ♦ Mortality:
  - – 10%

From: *Current Clinical Neurology: Handbook of Neurocritical Care*
Edited by: A. Bhardwaj, M. A. Mirski, and J. A. Ulatowski © Humana Press Inc., Totowa, NJ

Clinical Presentation

♦ Onset:
  – Acute: 24–72 h after exposure
  – Subacute: up to 20 d, sometimes even longer
♦ Duration:
  – If untreated, two weeks or more
♦ Symptoms:
  – Major: Fever, rigidity (lead pipe), elevated creatine kinase (CK)
  – Minor: autonomic instability (tachycardia, hyper or hypotension, diaphoresis); tachypnea; altered mental states (from confusion to coma); leukocytosis
  – Less reported: Seizure, opisthotonos, dystonia, chorea
♦ Laboratory Investigations:
  – Leukocytosis (>1000 iu/L)
  – Elevated liver function tests
  – Electrolyte imbalance
  – Normal lumbar puncture
♦ Associated adverse events:
  – Aspiration pneumonia
  – Circulatory collapse
  – Respiratory failure
  – Rhabdomyolysis
  – Acute renal failure
  – Pulmonary embolism
  – Heat stroke
  – Death

Differential Diagnosis

♦ Diagnosis:
  – Criteria for diagnosis is variable
  – Clinical research criteria include:
    • All major symptoms or
    • Two major and four minor symptoms
♦ Differential:
  – Central nervous system (CNS) infection
  – Lithium toxicity
  – 3,4'-methylenedioxymethamphetamine (ecstasy) toxicity
  – Serotonin syndrome
  – γ-aminobutyric acid (GABA)ergic agonist withdrawal
  – Monoamine oxidase (MAO) inhibitor use
  – Thyrotoxicosis

Table 1
Establishing Diagnosis of NMS

Management	Suggests inclusion of NMS as diagnosis	Suggests exclusion of NMS as diagnosis
1. History and physical	• History of offending agent(s) • Valid signs and symptoms • Absence of other possible diagnosis	• Lack of offending agent(s) • Atypical signs/symptoms (lack of fever rigidity, CK elevation; must consider alternate diagnosis)
2. Studies *Radiology:* head CT *Procedure:* lumbar puncture *Labs:* liver function tests, CK, complete blood count (CBC), blood urea nitrogen (BUN)/Cr, TSH/T4, toxicity screen, lithium level; cerebral spinal fluid (CSF) cell count with glucose, protein, cultures.	May include: • White blood cell (WBC) elevation • Metabolic acidosis • High CK (>1000 iu/L) • Mild elevated liver function tests • Absence of elevated lithium levels, toxicology screen positive, CNS infection, abnormal thyroid tests	• Abnormal CSF profile • Elevated lithium levels, toxicology screen positive for "ecstasy", abnormal thyroid tests • Normal CK, lack of fever, or rigidity

- Acute porphyria
- Tetany
- Akinetic mutism
- Lethal catatonia
- Rhabdomyolysis from other causes
- Neuroleptic induced heat stroke
- Malignant hyperthermia
- Central anticholinergic syndrome

Treatment

♦ Monitoring:
  - Airway
  - Forced vital capacity

- Vital signs for autonomic instability:
  - Tachycardia, tachypnea, hypertension, hypotension
- Fluid balance
- CK levels
- Aspiration risk
♦ Supportive:
  - Consider ICU monitoring
  - Aspiration precautions
  - Correct acidosis, consider sodium bicarbonate if $HCO_3 \leq 12–13$
  - Deep venous thrombosis (DVT) prophylaxis:
    - Heparin subcutaneous, graduated compression stockings (TEDs), sequential compression devices
  - Aggressive IV hydration; prevent rhabdomyolysis-induced renal failure
  - Withdrawal of offending agent
  - Avoid all dopamine antagonists,including metoclopramide
  - Tapering of anticholinergics
  - Reinstating dopaminergic agents. If was withdrawn
  - Aggressive cooling to normothermia:
    - Cooling blanket, alcohol wipe down, fans, etc.
♦ Pharmacologic-limited clinical studies show bromocriptine and dantrolene may be effective in treatment of NMS. Dialysis is ineffective in removal of offending agents:
  - Bromocriptine: decreases duration and mortality:
    - Dose: 5mg PO or PNGT qid, to maximum of 45 mg a day.
    - Caution: may worsen pyschosis
  - Dantrolene: decreases duration and mortality:
    - Dose: 2–3 mg/kg/d. Initial load of 2 mg/kg. Total dose not to exceed 1 mg/kg/d
    - Caution: hepatotoxicity
  - Bromocriptine and dantrolene may be used in conjunction with one and another but there is no data to support increased effectiveness
♦ Second-line pharmacologic agents:
  - Benzodiazapines
  - Amantidine
  - Levodopa/carbidopa
  - Carbamazepine (2 cases)
♦ Second-line therapy:
  - Electroconvulsive therapy (ECT): may help fever, diaphoresis, level of consciousness

Key Points

♦ NMS is potentially life threatening. Airway and vital signs must be closely monitored

♦ CNS infection must ruled out in suspected patients

♦ Exposure to neuroleptics, typical or atypical, as well as any dopamine antagonist, such as metoclopramide, may trigger NMS

♦ Classic symptoms include "lead pipe" rigidity, fever, dysautonomia, and elevated CK

♦ Aggressive hydration will help avoid development of renal failure

♦ Bromocriptine and dantrolene have been found to reduce duration of symptoms and mortality

Suggested Reading

Adnet P, Lestavel P, and Krivosic-Horber R. Neuroleptic malignant syndrome. *Brit J Anesthes* 2000;85(1):129–135.

Gordon PH and Frucht SJ. Neuroleptic malignant syndrome in advanced Parkinson's disease. *Movement Disorders* 2001;16(5):960–974.

Gurrera RJ. Is neuroleptics malignant syndrome a neurogenic form of malignant hyperthermia? *Clin Neuropharm* 2002;25 (4):183–193.

Lappa A, Semeraro F, et al. Successful treatment of a complicated case of neuroleptics malignant syndrome. *Int Care Med* 2002;28:976–977.

Nishioka Y, Kohno S, et al. Acute renal failure in neuroleptics malignant syndrome. *Renal Failure* 2002;24(4):539–543.

Susman VL. Clinical management of neuroleptics malignant syndrome. *Psychiatry Quarterly* 2001;72(4):325–336.

22 Brain Death and Organ Donation

Chere M. Chase and Michael A. Williams

Basic Concepts

♦ For over 30 yr, there has been debate over different concepts of brain death, but there is a widely accepted and practiced standard of determining brain death by the whole brain death concept

♦ Using the whole brain death concept, brain death is defined as the irreversible absence of all brain function, including the brainstem

♦ Determination of brain death requires expert knowledge and diagnostic skills

♦ Organ donation is closely linked to brain death, and intensive care unit (ICU) teams have an important role in helping families consider organ donation

Background

♦ All 50 states in the United States and the District of Columbia have similar legal definitions of brain death (Uniform Definition of Death Act). There remain some state- and hospital-based differences in the process for determining brain death

♦ The American Academy of Neurology has published a practice parameter for the diagnosis of brain death in patients older than 18 yr

♦ Brain death can result from a wide variety of causes, including trauma (e.g., subdural or epidural hematomas, penetrating ballistic injury), infection (e.g., meningitis, encephalitis, abscess), vascular disease (e.g., aneurysmal or arterio-venous malformation [AVM]-associated subarachnoid hemorrhage [SAH], intracerebral hemorrhage [ICH], large cerebral infarction, dural sinus thrombosis),

From: *Current Clinical Neurology: Handbook of Neurocritical Care*
Edited by: A. Bhardwaj, M. A. Mirski, and J. A. Ulatowski © Humana Press Inc., Totowa, NJ

hypoxic-ischemic encephalopathy (e.g., cardiac arrest or drowning), obstructive hydrocephalus, tumor (with associated edema and herniation syndrome), and metabolic encephalopathy (e.g., cerebral edema associated with fulminant hepatic failure, profound hyponatremia, or rapidly-corrected hyperosmolar hyperglycemic coma)
♦ In most instances, brain death follows one of the cerebral herniation syndromes, and has occurred despite brain resuscitation attempts

Management

♦ A neurologist, neurosurgeon or a specially trained clinician should perform the brain death examination
♦ A reliable and standardized process for performing and documenting the brain death exam is recommended
  – First, the medical record, history, imaging studies, and laboratory values should be reviewed to determine whether the prerequisite conditions for brain death exist. The conditions are:
    • Evidence of catastrophic brain injury with deep coma
    • Absence of sedative, narcotic, hypnotic or anesthetic agents
    • Absence of intoxication with alcohol or other drugs
    • Absence of circulatory shock, defined as systolic blood pressure (SBP) <90 mmHg
    • Absence of neuromuscular blockade (paralytic agents)
    • Absence of de-efferenting syndromes, including neuromuscular disease (e.g., Guillain–Barré syndrome, myasthenia gravis), acute high cervical (C1–C5) myelopathy, or brain stem infarction with locked-in syndrome
    • Absence of hypothermia, defined as core temperature ≤32° C
    • Absence of metabolic derangements that can affect brain function, including hypo- or hyperglycemia, ketoacidosis, uremia, hepatic failure, hypernatremia, hyponatremia, hypercalcemia
  – The diagnosis of brain death in patient with coma of undetermined origin is difficult. There are no study guidelines to address the dilemma. However, if the patient meets the clinical criteria, has a prolonged period of observation (>24 h), and has no cerebral blood flow, and if confounding factors have been excluded, it is reasonable to make a diagnosis of brain death

Brain Death Examination

♦ Once it is determined that the pre-requisite conditions are met, the brain death examination can and should be performed

Table 1
Prerequisite Criteria for Brain Death Examination

Criteria	*Recommended ranges*
Evidence of catastrophic brain injury	Clinical or neuroimaging evidence
Blood Glucose	>60 and <400 mg/dL
Blood Pressure:	
Systolic blood pressure (SBP)	>90 mmHg
Diastolic blood pressure (DBP)	>40 mmHg
Heart Rate	>30/min
PCO_2	>35 and <45 Torr
Temperature	>32°C

♦ For adults, the demonstration of irreversible loss of brain function requires two brain death examinations that are usually six hours apart, or more. For children, particularly infants less than one year of age, this interval is frequently longer

♦ Documentation of both brain death examinations is essential and should be performed with great attention to detail

Cranial Nerve Examination

♦ Pupillary constriction to light (Cranial nerves II and III) should be checked in a dark room. Pupil diameter should be mid-range or dilated to begin. The reflex must be absent bilaterally

♦ Oculocephalic reflex (Cranial nerves III and VI) are assessed by holding the eyes open and gently rotating the head from side-to-side (doll's eyes test). If there is no movement of the eyes, the reflex is absent. This should *not* be performed if there is evidence of fracture or instability of the cervical spine

♦ Vestibulo-ocular reflex (Cranial nerves III, VI and VIII). Determine the ear canals are clear of obstruction, and the tympanic membranes are not ruptured. Using a 50–60 cc syringe with either an IV catheter or the tubing from a butterfly needle, with the needle cut off, for insertion into the ear canal, slowly instill 60 cc ice water into each ear canal separately. If there is no movement of the eyes, the reflex is absent

♦ Corneal reflex (Cranial nerves V and VII) can be tested with a drop of sterile saline or the wisp of a cotton swab to stimulate the cornea. If there is no blink (including absence of subtle lower lid movement), the reflex is absent

♦ Facial grimace (Cranial nerves V and VII) can be tested by pressing on the supraorbital ridge. If there is no facial grimace, the reflex is absent

♦ Cough/gag reflex (Cranial nerves IX and X). Pass a suction catheter via the endotracheal tube to stimulate the carina. If there is no cough or gag, the reflex is absent. Side-to-side or up-and-down jiggling of the endotracheal (ET) tube is an insufficient stimulus for the brain death examination

– Additionally, a cotton swab can be gently inserted into the nasopharynx via the nostril, taking care to direct the swab posteriorly toward the pharynx, and not superiorly toward the cribriform plate. If there is no gag, cough, or facial grimace, the reflex is absent

Motor Examination

♦ There should be no spontaneous or reflex motor responses

♦ For the determination of brain death, an intense noxious stimulus is justified to demonstrate absence of response, but it is not justifiable to use instruments (e.g., clamps, hemostats), or other objects that would physically harm the patient. Because the absence of motor responses is best determined by assessing movement of the arms, it is preferable to apply the stimulus on the trunk or head, rather than on the fingertips so as not to hold the limb being observed. Adequate stimuli include pressure on the supraorbital ridge, stylomastoid process, clavicle or sternum, or pinching the trapezius. Flexion, extension, and localizing responses must be absent. Movements of spinal cord origin occasionally occur, and may be difficult to distinguish from cortical motor movements. It is often advisable to have a colleague examine this movement independently to confirm the spinal origin

♦ There should be no autonomic response to the application of painful stimuli or to vagal stimuli. The electroechocardiogram (EKG) monitor can be set up so that there is an audible tone with every cardiac cycle so that changes in rate or rhythm or more easily detected. When applying a painful stimulus, there should be no cardiac acceleration. With compression of the ocular globes, there should be no bradycardia

Apnea Test

♦ There is variation in practice, but because the apnea test can result in hypotension, hypercapnea and hypoxia with lethal arrhythmias, our practice is to perform the apnea test only once, at the time of the second exam. The rationale of the apnea test is apneic oxygenation, that is to allow the $PaCO_2$ to rise to a sufficient level that respiration should occur, but not to allow hypoxia

- Suggested prerequisites for the apnea test are the same as for the brain-death examination in general, but with the addition of:
  - Normocapnea (PaCO2 35–45 Torr)
  - Normoxemia (Pre-oxygenation at FiO_2 1.0 can help to delay or prevent hypoxia)
  - Adequate physiologic monitoring is present, including continuous arterial blood pressure measurement, EKG and arrhythmia monitoring, and pulse oximetry
- An arterial blood gas (ABG) immediately before the apnea test should confirm normocapnea and adequate oxygenation
- Apneic oxygenation requires inserting a tube into the ET tube in order to deliver O_2 at the level of the carina. We recommend using a tracheal suction catheter for this purpose, as it is designed to go through an ET tube without occluding it. If there is a thumb hole on the suction catheter, it should be occluded or taped. The suction catheter is then connected to O_2 tubing. The ventilator tubing is removed from the ET tube, and the suction catheter, with O_2 at a rate of 4–6 lpm, is inserted to the carina. It is not sufficient to perform apneic oxygenation by changing the ventilator mode to continuous positive airway pressure (CPAP), or by placing a T-piece on the ET tube. Because of the dead space of the ET tube and airway, as well as the fact that gas will flow via the path of least resistance (i.e., through the ventilator tubing or the T-piece rather than into the ET tube), neither of these methods directs O_2 to the carina or nearby alveoli, and hypoxia will occur much rapidly
- Apneic oxygenation should be performed long enough to allow the $PaCO_2$ to reach 60 Torr or more. Depending on the patient's basal metabolic rate, this can take as long as 15 min. Thus, as long as the blood pressure (BP), cardiac rhythm, and SaO_2 are stable, it is often wise to wait for ABG results before reconnecting the ventilator, because if the ventilator has already been reconnected and the $PaCO_2$ is then discovered to be too low, the entire apnea test may need to be repeated. One option is to obtain ABGs at 5-min intervals
- For patients with chronic obstructive pulmonary disease (COPD) who have chronic hypercapnea, a $PaCO_2$ rise of 20 Torr above baseline is commonly accepted, provided the initial $PaCO_2$ for the apnea test approximates the patient's premorbid baseline $PaCO_2$

– Because the apnea test requires observation of the absence of respiratory effort, the examiner must stay at the bedside for the entire duration of the apnea test. Many examiners will place their hand on the patient's chest in order to palpate respiratory movement. The examiner's presence is also required to respond to the potential complications of the apnea test

– Particularly for patients with lung injury or disease, hypoxia may occur during apneic oxygenation before the $PaCO_2$ goal is reached. In such circumstances, an ABG should be obtained before reconnecting the ventilator, so that the PaO_2 and $PaCO_2$ can be documented. Although there is no standard for using PaO_2 as a criterion for determining absence of respiratory drive in brain death determination, there is established physiologic literature on the effects of hypoxia on respiratory drive. In these uncommon circumstances, provided that all other components of the brain-death examination confirm brain death, it may be justified to conclude that the absence of hypoxic respiratory drive is consistent with brain death. This rationale and the ABG results should be clearly documented, and discussion or confirmation with a colleague may be advisable

– The apnea test should be terminated and the ventilator reconnected if:

• There is any cough, gasp, or respiratory effort. If this occurs, the patient is not brain dead

• Hemodynamic instability cannot be managed with vasopressors or fluids. If the apnea test must be stopped for this reason, obtain an ABG before reconnecting the ventilator. If the ABG results do not support absence of respiratory effort, then a confirmatory test, such as cerebral blood flow studies, angiography, or electroencephalogram (EEG) may need to be performed

• The $PaCO_2$ is >60 torr (>8 kPa) or higher in the case of COPD

• If there is no respiratory movement during apneic oxygenation, then brainstem respiratory drive is absent

• If the apnea test is the final component of the brain death examination, then this result confirms brain death. *Note:* The apnea test performed in the absence of the other components of the brain death examination is insufficient to determine brain death

♦ Ancillary testing for brain-death determination is optional, and there is variation in practice patterns. Radionuclide cerebral blood flow studies and cerebral angiography are commonly used, and have the advantage that they can be performed after a single clinical examination consistent with brain death has been performed. If these studies demonstrate absence of intracranial blood flow or perfusion, they confirm brain death. If long-acting anesthetics (e.g., pentobarbital) have been used to treat intracranial pressure, clinical brain death testing cannot be performed, and blood flow studies are advisable. Transcranial Doppler sonography is widely available, but is not considered sufficient by itself to confirm brain death. While EEG is widely available, it represents only cortical function, and therefore brainstem function should be assessed separately

Organ Donation
Basic Concepts

♦ Transplantation of tissues and solid organs is an accepted therapy for many debilitating and life-threatening illness. However, the number of donated organs in the United States is significantly less than needed for patients awaiting transplantation

♦ United States federal regulations and many state laws require all institutions to designate a person or persons to present families of every deceased patient the option of organ and tissue donation

♦ In the United States, organ and tissue procurement is performed by federally regulated and funded organ procurement organizations (OPOs). OPO staff, including transplantation coordinators and family advocates, are involved in the process of requesting organ donation

Epidemiology

♦ By the end of 1999, the Organ Procurement and Transplantation Network identified 72,110 patients who required organ donation. While on the waiting list, 8.5% of these patients died

♦ The number of potential organ donors (brain-dead patients meeting medical eligibility criteria) in the United States is 8000–15,000 annually, but there are only about 5000–6000 donors per year

  – The unrealized donor potential has three major sources:

   • An estimated 25% of the families of eligible donors are not given the option of donation because the donors were not identified or the healthcare team did not approach the family

- Donor-eligible African-American families are only half as likely to be offered the option of donation as donor-eligible white families
- There is a low consent rate among families offered organ donation as an option

Management

♦ The care of brain-dead patients and their families, including the request for organ donation, should be considered a special variant of end-of-life (EOL) care

♦ The process, sequence, timing, and coordination of family meetings and communication influence families' willingness to consent to organ donation. The consent rate is higher when persons have been specially trained in this process, and when the ICU team and OPO staff support one another

♦ Physicians play an important role in organ donation by supporting the presentation of the option of donation to all families, and to work closely with the OPO staff

♦ A "decoupled" approach to the organ donation request is frequently used. Decoupling implies that the discussion of organ donation occurs separately from (and after) notification of patient's death. In many situations, decoupling takes the form of the ICU team first telling the family that the patient has been pronounced dead, and then returning later with the OPO transplantation coordinator to begin consideration of organ donation

♦ Organ donation cannot occur without OPO involvement. By virtue of their role in caring for patients who are brain dead and may be potential organ donors, ICU physicians and staff play an important and irreplaceable part in the process of organ donation and transplantation. ICU staff should notify OPOs of all patients who are expected to die, and federal regulations in the United States now require that this referral be made. Criteria vary from institution to institution for contacting the OPO; however, a Glasgow Coma Scale (GCS) ≤5 is commonly used. This allows the OPO staff time to review the patient's case and discuss it with the ICU team

♦ Contrary to the often-heard disparagement of OPO staff as "vultures" waiting to swoop down for organs, OPO staff nearly always have prior experience caring for families of dying patients (e.g., as nurses, physician assistants, or social workers), and are as dedicated to caring for potential donors' families as ICU staff are. In fact, one of the most important variables emerging as an influence on consent for organ donation is the amount of time the OPO staff spends with the family

Organ Donation After Cardiac Death (Non-Heartbeating Donation)

♦ Patients declared dead by cardiopulmonary criteria can also be suitable candidates for organ donation (organ donation after cardiac death [ODCD])

♦ ODCD can be uncomfortable for ICU teams to consider, as it brings together EOL decision making, withdrawal of life-sustaining therapies, death, and organ donation in an uncommon circumstance. The potential for conflict of interest is of most concern to many ICU physicians and staff

♦ ODCD occurs when a patient, or more commonly, the patient's family decides with the ICU team to withdraw life-sustaining therapies. Occasionally, families will ask whether organ donation is possible, and in some ICUs, families are routinely presented this option

♦ The physiologic and ethical issues involved include, but are not limited to:

   – ODCD requires continuation of life-sustaining therapy until the resources for organ procurement (e.g., OPO involvement, OR availability) are arranged

   – For ODCD to occur, the patient's death should occur within 60 min of withdrawal of life-sustaining therapies. Otherwise the duration of warm ischemia may be too long for the transplanted organs to be viable

   – The location of withdrawal of life-sustaining therapies and death may be the ICU or the operating room, depending on individual institutional circumstances and policy

   – The physician pronouncing death must not be from the team procuring organs

   – The duration of pulselessness necessary to declare death is based on the concept that the duration should be long enough that cardiac autoresuscitation is not possible. This time interval varies from hospital to hospital, and is as short as two minutes and as long as from eight to ten min

   – If the patient does not die in time for ODCD to occur, the patient should return from the operating room to the ICU, or to another hospital location so that palliative care can be continued

Key Points

♦ Brain death should be diagnosed by a neurologist, neurosurgeon, or other specially trained physicians

♦ Irreversible absence of all brain function, including the brainstem is needed

♦ Ancillary tests and prolonged observation and repeated examinations may be necessary

♦ Organ donation candidacy should be considered for all brain dead patients.

♦ Families should be given the option by specially trained individuals after adequate time to decouple events leading to death

Suggested Reading

Wijdicks EFM, ed. Brain Death: A Clinical Guide.. Philadelphia, PA: Lippincott Williams and Wilkins; 2001.

Committee on Non-Heart-Beating Transplantation II: The Scientific and Ethical Basis for Practice and Protocols, Division of Health Care Services, Institute of Medicine. Non-Heart-Beating Organ Transplantation. Practice and Protocols. Washington DC: National Academy Press; 2000

Ethics Committee, American College of Critical Care Medicine, Society of Critical Care Medicine. Recommendations for nonheart-beating organ donation. *Crit Care Med* 2001; 29:1826–1831

Quality Standards Subcommittee of the American Academy of Neurology. Practice parameters for determining brain death in adults. *Neurology* 1995;45:1012–1014.

Siminoff LA, Gordon N, Hewlett J, and Arnold RM. Factors influencing families' consent for donation of solid organs for transplantation. *JAMA* 2001;286:71–77.

Van Norman GA. A matter of life and death: What an anesthesiologist should know about the medical, legal, and ethical aspects of declaring brain death. *Anesthesiology* 1999;91:275–287.

Wang MY, Wallace P, and Gruen JP. Brain death documentation: analysis and issues. *Neurosurgery* 2002;51:731–736

Wijdicks, EFM. Determining brain death in adults. *Neurology* 1995:45:1003–1011.

Williams MA, Lipsett P, Rushton CH, et al. The physician's role in discussing organ donation with families. Council on Scientific Affairs, American Medical Association. *Crit Care Med* 2003;31:1568 –1573

Williams MA, and Suarez JI. Brain death determination in adults: More than meets the eye. *Crit Care Med* 1997;25:1787–1788.

23 Ethical Issues and Withdrawal of Life-Sustaining Therapies

Chere M. Chase and Michael A. Williams

Basic Concepts

♦ The foundation of ethics is the nature of morals and the specific moral perspective that people have when they relate to others
♦ Ethical frameworks are used to set standards of conduct (normative behaviors) by which members of a profession are governed and judged
♦ Caring for the sick, especially critically ill patients, requires constant attention to ethical frameworks and processes to support decision making in varying clinical, cultural, and professional environments where persons with different moral perspectives must make decisions together
♦ "End of life (EOL) decision making" in the intensive care unit (ICU) involves decisions to initiate, continue, limit, or withdraw therapies, and includes resuscitation status, palliative care, and withdrawal of life sustaining therapies

Historical Perspective

♦ As a result of the medical contributions of Dr. Peter Safar and colleagues in cardiopulmonary resuscitation (CPR) and the advent of ICU therapies, persons who would otherwise have died under previous standards of care survived. Medical decisions surrounding therapy, resuscitation, or withdrawal of therapies were presumably less complicated then. The ethical and legal framework was less well developed. With the prevailing approach at the time, physicians decided what was best for patients and which therapies would or would not be used. This is known as paternalism

From: *Current Clinical Neurology: Handbook of Neurocritical Care*
Edited by: A. Bhardwaj, M. A. Mirski, and J. A. Ulatowski © Humana Press Inc., Totowa, NJ

♦ Along with emergence of biomedical ethics as an academic field, there was important legal and court recognition of the autonomy of patients and their families (e.g., In re Quinlan. 355 A.2d 647 [NJ] 1976). Health care professionals (HCPs), patients and their families have struggled with decisions and practices involved in initiating, continuing, or discontinuing life-sustaining therapies (LST), particularly in the ICU. Over the last 25 yr, the role of patient self-determination (autonomy) and the right of families or surrogates to make proxy decisions for patients who lack decision making capacity has shifted the dynamic of practice toward a model known as shared decision making

♦ By its very nature, the shared decision-making model incorporates views and values of patients, families, ICU physicians and nurses, and other HCPs caring for patients. While there is often consensus regarding decisions and care, there are also many times when the views and values of the participants differ, sometimes with conflict as a result

♦ Recent studies have shown the number of deaths in ICUs after withdrawal of life sustaining measures is increasing such that 70–90% of ICUs deaths occur after a decision to limit therapy

♦ Planning for severe illness or dying (advance care planning) has been a focus of many laws (e.g., Patient Self Determination Act), regulations (e.g., Joint Commission on Accreditation of Healthcare Organizations [JCAHO]), medical specialty societies, and health care institutions for over 10 yr

   – As a result, some patients have been previously counseled about EOL decisions, and have indicated their values and preferences concerning medical treatment and palliative care. It is estimated that no more than 10–15% of hospitalized patients have advance directives (ADs) or living wills

   – Some patients have a legally designated surrogate—proxy or health care agent—with durable power of attorney for health care decisions, and some states have laws that indicate who may make these decisions for patients who have not made such a designation. The majority of the time, patients' wishes are not well known, and it falls to ICU physicians and nurses to undertake conversations with patients and their families concerning the patient's values and preferences in the process of medical decision making

♦ There is significant variability in the approach to withdrawal of life sustaining therapies within countries and among cultures. The increasing trend for patients to travel to other countries for their health care means that ethical framework and cultural underpinnings ICU teams use for EOL decisions may not match those of patients and families with different cultural perspectives

Management: An Overview

♦ Critically ill patients often benefit from intensive care, with resulting survival and quality outcomes. When ICU therapies are started, particularly for acute illnesses of uncertain outcome, the benefits of therapies and the chances of survival with an acceptable outcome (i.e., beneficience) usually prevail over any risk of discomfort, pain, or complications of therapies. Thus, patients, families, and ICU teams accept the burdens of the interventions in hopes of curing patients

♦ Critically ill patients can die despite the best efforts of ICU teams. Sometimes critically ill patients survive with outcomes that are widely viewed as poor (e.g., vegetative state)

  – The ICU team's approach to these circumstances, particularly to dying patients, has the power to make the critical illness or death either a memorable experience, or a miserable experience for the patient and family

♦ There is a constant tension between curative therapies and palliative therapies

  – In many instances, it seems that curative therapies are pursued alone until the ICU team decides "nothing more can be done." This model (cure..cure..cure..."ooops!"...palliative care) often catches families unaware or unprepared for the fact that the patient has always been at risk of dying. When families are unprepared, resistance and conflict can easily arise

♦ Palliative therapies have no prerequisite that patients must be dying

  – Palliative care is more than EOL care. It is "a comprehensive approach to treating serious illness that focuses on physical, psychological, spiritual, and social needs of patients. The goal is to achieve the best quality of life achievable by relieving suffering, controlling pain and symptoms, and enabling maximum functional capacity"

  – Curative and palliative therapies can and should be pursued in parallel. There should be a continuum consistent with the fact that patients and families do not suddenly switch from hope for survival and cure to acceptance of death and comfort measures. Even patients undergoing extreme therapies may also be in need of palliative therapies. The aim is to provide a balance of curative and

palliative therapies that matches patients' needs. The proportion of
curative and palliative therapies should change as the patient's
condition changes

♦ Health care professionals should recognize the effect of time on
their ability to meet patients' needs. This also affects the ability of
patients and families to comprehend the patients' condition, and to
respond both cognitively and emotionally. In ICUs, daily routines are
often hurried, and ICU teams can experience seeing critically ill
patients and making rapid decisions as virtually mundane. There is
often a mismatch between the time that HCPs need to make decisions
and the time which patients and families require

♦ Most agree that EOL decision-making requires careful and sensitive discussion, deliberation and exploration with patients and families. Physicians must be willing to devote the time necessary to
accomplish this

  – The process of shared decision-making requires frequent conversations between ICU team, patient, and family to identify and
  reassess the patient's condition, goals of care, response to therapies, and recommendations for further treatment. It is a mistake to
  believe that a single conversation suffices
  – Due to unfamiliarity with ICUs and the emotional stress associated with their circumstances, patients and families will usually
  not hear everything they are told in a family meeting. If the family
  is crying or appears stressed, stop talking and wait a few moments
  – Do not mistake an initial lack of understanding as either denial
  or intellectual shortcoming. Patience is vital. Information may
  have to be shared more than once
  – Be particularly attentive to avoid the use of ICU jargon and
  slang when talking to families. It is wise to ask whether you can
  explain anything better or differently for them
  – It is especially helpful to take an interdisciplinary approach to
  family meetings, including physician, nurse, hospital chaplain, or
  social worker

♦ A major risk in ICUs is that multiple members of the ICU team, or
multiple consultants will speak with the patient and family independently, rather than in a coordinated fashion. The inevitable result is
mixed messages to the family, with potential for confusion, anger,
focus on minor details rather than the "big picture", and so-called
splitting behaviors. It is the responsibility of the ICU team and consultants to reach consensus when possible, and respectfully identify

Table 1
Template for End-of-Life Decision-Making

As soon as you realize there is a chance a patient may die or have a poor prognosis, you should set up a meeting with the patient, family or surrogate

Whenever possible, involve another health professional, such as a nurse, social worker, or pastor. Plan the meeting with them

Meet in private. Tell the patient and family why the meeting has been scheduled

Discuss the possibility of death frankly and sensitively. Be prepared for their emotional responses and allow them to be expressed

Attempt to learn about the patient's preferences and values so that these can guide medical decisions

Explain treatment options and the range of outcomes, and address palliative care options

Make a recommendation based on your integrated understanding of the patient's preferences and the medical situation

Allow the patient or family to make decisions

After they make their decision, tell them what actions will occur as a result

If the decision is to continue therapy, then establish a time to meet with them again and repeat the process

If there is a failure to agree on the care plan, either between physicians and families, or amongst family members, the guidance of an ethics committee may helpful

Adapted from **Williams, MA.**;2002:9–12.

differences of opinion when necessary, *before* speaking with the patient or family:

– An important limitation of the perspective of many ICU team members in EOL decision making is that they do not usually see patients beyond their ICU stay. Thus, they may not have the experience of other team members (e.g., surgeons and other physicians) who provide longitudinal care. These HCPs have seen similar patients throughout their entire episode of care (i.e., after they leave the ICU), and may have a different perspective on the possibility of attaining the patient's desired outcomes

♦ The decision-making model includes regular assessment of the patient's response to treatment in light of goals of care, which are often long-term and global goals described in terms of life, death, and degree of acceptable impairment or disability

- Thus, the ICU team is often asked to use short-term response to therapy to predict, with varying degrees of certainty and uncertainty, whether the patient's desired long-term outcomes can be attained. The ICU team should disclose its sources of information (e.g.. literature or experience with similar patients) and the strength of the information when making recommendations

◆ If HCPs think the patient's response to therapy means that the goals of care are not attainable, then they should explain this empathetically, and recommend focusing more effort on the palliative goals of care, and less on the curative goals

◆ The phrase "there's nothing more that we can do" is utterly incorrect

- Even when curative therapies are no longer effective, there is much care that can be continued—palliative care
- Among other things, the palliative-care strategy helps prevent families from feeling as if they are being abandoned when the patient is dying, and may help members of the ICU team avoid feeling as if they are not meeting the needs of patients and families as death approaches

◆ The ICU team and support staff (e.g.. hospital chaplains or social workers) should inquire and prepare for relevant cultural expectations regarding the process of dying, handling the body after death, views about autopsy and organ donation, and cultural norms of grieving

Management: Patient Needs

◆ The focus of palliative care and EOL care includes alleviating suffering from physical, emotional, social and spiritual stress

◆ Patients' fears center mainly around:
- Pain and dyspnea
- Loss of dignity and respect, both before and after the dying process
- Loss of control (mental or bodily)
- Loss of the opportunity to say good-bye, make amends, or to be with family
- Fear that cultural expectations and concerns will not be met

Management: Family Needs

◆ Families' fears are similar to those of patients. Additional concerns may include:
- Fear of exclusion or separation from the patient
- Fear of not being able to explain death and dying to children, or to meet their emotional needs if someone they love is dying

Table 2
The Ten Most Important Needs of Families
of Critically Ill Dying Patients

1. To be with the person
2. To be helpful to the dying person
3. To be informed of the dying person's changing condition.
4. To understand what is being done to the patient and why
5. To be assured of the patient's comfort
6. To be comforted
7. To ventilate emotions
8. To be assured that their decisions were right
9. To find meaning in the dying of their loved one
10. To be fed, hydrated, and rested

Adapted from **Truog RD, et al.**;2002:2332–2348.

♦ Additional considerations include:
  – Arranging for a private room
  – Involving the hospital chaplain or bereavement counselor
  – Liberalized visitation, including children and extended family
  – Support for important rituals, including music, prayer, and
  bathing or preparation of the patient's body

Management: Needs of the Clinical Team

♦ All members of the health care team should play active roles in
the EOL care. These roles should be determined in advance
♦ ICU attending physicians should be role models by leading the
ICU team in the discussion and provision of palliative care, as they
can create continuity in the quality of the care and reinforce the
importance of integrating curative and palliative care to patients, their
families, students and residents, and the ICU staff
  – In one example of role modeling that could be considered
  "lacking", 36% of Society of Critical Care Medicine (SCCM)
  physicians who order extubation said that they do not personally
  remove the endotracheal tube; they have the nurse or respiratory
  therapist extubate. Those physicians' choices probably reflect their
  degree of comfort with EOL care and withdrawal of life sustaining
  interventions
  – There must be administrative and institutional commitment for
  critical care, palliative care, and EOL care, including the resources
  to provide this care

– The ICU team members can benefit from a protected forum in which to express their feelings and concerns, especially for "challenging cases". A standard debriefing process to review and discuss the EOL care of each patient may result in improved care processes for the ICU as a whole

Guidelines

♦ Consensus guidelines on EOL care in the intensive care unit are available. Regrettably, there is significant variability in the manner in which EOL care is provided in ICUs

♦ Most would agree that life-sustaining interventions include invasive monitoring or procedures, administration of vasopressors and other medications, laboratory studies, and radiographic studies. However, the status of artificial hydration and nutrition (AHN) is still debated

– Some consider AHN as life-sustaining therapies because they require the use of mechanical pumps or gravity feed to administer via catheter

– Others consider AHN more fundamental, and not "therapies" by virtue of their strong symbolism and connection to nurturing, love and sustenance

♦ Although beyond the scope of this chapter, palliative care is more than just the provision of narcotics or sedatives, and is quite distinct from calling "the pain service" to manage this care. In settings where palliative care consultants are available, invite their involvement early. They can provide important guidance to the ICU team, and support and reassurance to patients and families

♦ Although it may seem counterintuitive, withdrawal of certain life-sustaining therapies, in particular contexts, may result in more pain or discomfort than if they were retained. Generally speaking, this is more likely to occur with conscious rather than unconscious patients. This possibility should be considered and discussed among the health care team and with the patient and family

♦ The judicious use of analgesic and anti-anxiolytic medications to relieve pain and symptoms associate with dying is advocated by the American Academy of Neurology and the Society for Critical Care Medicine, provided the intent is to address pain and symptoms, and not to cause or hasten death

– However, the fear of hastening or assisting death, or even the appearance of doing so, leaves many health care teams divided on the use of these agents. Studies have shown that opioids and

Table 3
Possible Adverse Symptoms of Forgoing Specific Therapies

System	Intervention	Effect of withdrawal
Cardiovascular	Vasopressors	Hypotension with resulting tachycardia
	Intra-aortic balloon pump	Decreased coronary perfusion (angina)
	Cardiac pacemaker	Bradycardia, decreased cardiac output (symptomatic heart failure)
Pulmonary	Oxygen	Sympathetic discharge Air hunger and increased respiratory drive
	Mechanical ventilation	Hypercapnea, increased respiratory drive, coma
	Positive end-expiratory pressure	Ventilation-perfusion mismatching, hypoxia
	Extubation	Potential for stridor, gagging, airway obstruction
Renal	Dialysis	Acidosis, uremia, fluid overload, delirium
Neurologic	External cerebrospinal fluid drainage	Increased intracranial pressure, coma, posturing, changes in respiratory pattern (spontaneous hyperventilation or gasping)
Nutritional	Nutrition and hydration	Lipolysis, ketosis, dehydration

Adapted from **Truog RD et al.**;2002:2332-2348.

benzodiazepines used as part of withdrawal of life-sustaining therapy *do not* hasten death

♦ The ethical principle of "double effect" is based on the premise that the intent of symptom management is to ease suffering, and that in the context of deteriorating homeostatic physiological functions associated with dying, the effect on cardiorespiratory function is unavoidable and is ethically permissible

♦ Careful attention should be placed to the manner in which orders for narcotics and sedatives are written and documented. The order should indicate measurable signs or symptoms (e.g., appearance of pain, anxiety, or dyspnea) by which the nursing staff will administer the medication or titrate its dose. If the signs or symptoms are controlled, then the dose need not be increased or administered

- More to the point, such orders should not be written with a physiologic goal that would appear to have the intent of harming or causing death (such as "keep RR < 8 or mean arterial pressure <70")
- At the same time, the dosing or titration interval should match the pharmacologic profile of each medication so that if the patient is experiencing symptoms, the medication can be administered in a timely manner. The aim is to be sure the patient's symptoms are not left untreated by virtue of "having to wait" for a dosing interval that is inappropriate for the patient's needs and the onset and duration of the medication's effects
- Starting doses and titration schedules are merely guidelines. Since many patients in the ICU have already been exposed to sedative and analgesic therapies and developed a tolerance for them, these agents should be titrated to effect
- The Ethics Committee of the SCCM recommends "anticipatory dosing" of analgesia or sedation in the context of withdrawal of therapies, particularly extubation or withdrawal of ventilatory support. Rather than wait, or react to the appearance of distress, the aim is to anticipate it and administer adequate doses of sedation or analgesia (within the framework of the principle of double effect and the intent to relieve symptoms) shortly before the therapies are removed. A two- to three-fold increase of hourly dose may be necessary for conscious patients. Unconscious patients are less likely to experience distress at the time of extubation, and should be treated on an individualized basis

♦ Extubation is an important concern in the withdrawal of life sustaining therapies

- As many as 15% of critical care physicians reveal that do not feel comfortable with withdrawal of mechanical ventilation
- There are two commonly used methods of withdrawal of mechanical ventilation. One is "terminal extubation", which involves removal of the endotracheal tube, usually with appropriate administration of anxiolytics and narcotic analgesics to address dyspnea
- The second is known as "terminal weaning" which involves gradually reducing the FiO_2 or the ventilatory rate while watching to see if the patient takes over spontaneous respiration. This wean is performed over minutes to days as determined by the clinician

- Approximately 33% of SCCM physicians choose terminal weaning, 13% extubation, and the remainder do both
- Extubation carries the potential benefit of relieving the discomfort of the ET tube, and allowing conscious patients the opportunity to speak with their family. It also can be scheduled for a particular time, and it is completed in a short period of time. Potential burdens are that patients with copious oropharyngeal secretions, or those with impaired pharyngeal and laryngeal control may gasp, gag, or have stridor after extubation
- Physicians who favor "terminal weaning" often feel that this approach is less like "killing", as it gives patients the opportunity to breathe spontaneously, and if they do not, then they have died of respiratory insufficiency rather than extubation
- Another option to consider is immediate withdrawal of ventilatory support without extubation. For patients who are unconscious, there is no burden from being unable to speak, as they already cannot, and there is potential benefit in preventing the appearance of stridor or gasping. Although it is possible that spontaneous breathing may last longer because of the patent airway, the increased airway resistance offered by the endotracheal (ET) tube may counter this effect
- If done with patient comfort in mind and performed in an expeditious and timely fashion, any of these methods are acceptable. It is advisable to discuss the palliative care goals of extubation with the patient and family, and to take the approach that is most appropriate for them
- Similarly, the use of sedation for withdrawal of ventilatory support from conscious patients should be guided by the patient's goals. Some wish the opportunity to speak with their family and friends, and others do not want awareness of any pain or discomfort as they die
♦ The use of neuromuscular blockade (paralytic agents) deserves special mention
- If these agents are not part of a patient's therapeutic regimen prior to extubation or withdrawal of ventilatory support, then their use is inappropriate, as they address no palliative care need
- If these agents are part of a patient's therapeutic regimen (e.g., tetanus, acute respiratory distress syndrome [ARDS]), then their need should be assessed by attempting to withdraw them or reduce their dose *prior* to withdrawal of ventilatory support, and watching for evidence of painful muscular contraction or dyspnea caused by muscular rigidity

- In those *rare* circumstances in which it appears that withdrawal
of neuromuscular blockade would result in pain or suffering, consultation with the hospital Ethics Consultation Service is strongly
recommended

Controversies

♦ Research involving patients with ADs or do-not-resuscitate
(DNR) status. Critical care specialists are relying more and more
on evidence-based medicine to guide innovative therapies to save
persons who would otherwise die. However, the clinical research
needed to generate the evidence base in the critically ill patient
population has become more challenging with increased numbers
of patients and families making end of life decisions

  - Therefore, in academic medical centers, the decision to conduct
  clinical research involving critically ill patients is frequently in
  potential conflict with the clinical mission to make treatment decisions in the best interest of individual patients
  - It is both possible and desirable to consider patients with
  advance directives and DNR status eligible to participate in critical
  care research. To do otherwise could bias the study sample and
  unjustly exclude the opportunity to participate in research from a
  significant group of patients. If a research intervention is more
  effective than standard therapy, then fewer subjects in the study
  group will reach the point of invoking the AD

♦ Futility. The concept of medical futility is a controversial topic and
there is no national consensus on its definition or scope.
Occasionally, HCPs view specific treatments that are being provided,
requested, or considered as ineffective or futile. This can include
treatments that were begun with the expectation of improvement, and
that subsequently do not produce the desired outcome and cannot
prevent the deterioration of the patient's condition. Physicians are not
obligated to provide treatment that is considered medically ineffective
or futile

♦ However, physicians should recognize that only a small percent of
patients are sick enough to invoke "futility"

♦ In addition, for most HCPs, defining medical futility can be
extremely difficult. Disagreement between nurses and doctors with
respect to futility of medical interventions frequently exists

  - As a general rule, the physiologic effectiveness of a particular
  therapy and the prognosticators of achieving the goals of care
  should be considered together when attempting to define futility

♦ Intensive care unit teams are obliged to inform patients and families if they believe therapy is futile. Families who have been prepared for the possibility of death or poor outcome may be more willing to accept the ICU team's pronouncement. For those families who do not accept this news or the recommendation to limit or withdraw therapies, the ICU team is obliged to offer them further time and consideration (due process approach)

– It is not appropriate to make a unilateral determination of futility, or to order limitation or withdrawal of therapies without the family's involvement

– The Ethics Committee should be involved, however it is important to understand that their role is *not* to "tell the family that this is futile." It is to review the ethical issues of the case and offer guidance to the health care team about the ethical permissibility of available options

– In circumstances when the issue of futility cannot be resolved, an important option is to give the patient and family the chance to request and receive care by another ICU or hospital. Therapies should be continued while the family is pursuing this option

Key Points

♦ 70–90% of deaths in the ICU are associated with limitation or withdrawal of life-sustaining therapies
♦ Decisions on ending life-sustaining therapies are not unilateral and require disclosure and education of patient family, health care professionals
♦ All health care professionals and a family support structure (e.g., social worker, clergy) are important members of the team approach to withdrawal of life support
♦ Once a decision on withdrawal of life support has been made, management focuses on measures addressing comfort and dignity
♦ Institutional ethics committees may help when disagreement persists

Suggested Reading

Abbott KH, Sago JG, Breen CM, Abernethy AP, and Tulsky JA. Families looking back: One year after discussion of withdrawal or withholding of life-sustaining support. *Crit Care Med* 2001;29:197–201.
Brody II, Campbell MI, Faber-Langendoen K, et al. Withdrawing intensive life sustaining treatment - Recommendations for compassionate clinical management. *N England J Med* 1997;336:652–657.

Buckman, R. *How to Break Bad News: A Guide for Health Care Professionals.* Baltimore, Maryland: Johns Hopkins University Press; 1992.

Council on Ethical and Judicial Affairs, American Medical Association. Medical futility in end-of-life care. Report of the Council on Ethical and Judicial Affairs. *JAMA* 1999;281:937–994.

Curtis JR and Rubenfeld GD, eds. *Managing Death in the Intensive Care Unit. The Transition from Cure to Comfort.* New York: Oxford University Press; 2001.

Ethics and Humanities Subcommittee, American Academy of Neurology. Palliative care in neurology. *Neurology* 1996;46:870–872

Rushton CH, Williams MA, and Sabatier KH. The integration of palliative care and critical care: one vision, one voice. *Crit Care Nurs Clin North Am* 2002;14:133–140.

Truog RD, Cist AFM, Brackett SE, et al. Recommendations for end-of-life care in the intensive care unit: The Ethics Committee of the Society of Critical Care Medicine. *Crit Care Med* 2002;29:2332–2348

Williams, MA. The role of neurologists in end-of-life decision making and care. In: *Current Therapy of Neurologic Disease,* 6th ed (Johnson RT, Griffin JW, and McArthur JC, eds.), St. Louis: Mosby;2002: 9–12.

Williams MA and C Haywood, Jr. Critical care research on patients with advance directives and do-not-resuscitate status: Ethical challenges for clinician-investigators. *Crit Care Med* 2003; 31(Suppl):S167–S171.

http://www.lastacts.org/

http://www.eperc.mcw.edu

Index